10.75

SIGFRID FREGERT

MANUAL OF
CONTACT DERMATITIS

SECOND EDITION

On behalf of the

INTERNATIONAL CONTACT DERMATITIS
RESEARCH GROUP

H-J. Bandmann (Munich, West Germany), C. D. Calnan (London, England), E. Cronin (London, England), S. Fregert (Lund, Sweden), N. Hjorth (Copenhagen, Denmark), J-M. Lachapelle (Bruxelles, Belgium), H. I. Maibach (San Francisco, Calif., USA), K. E. Malten (Nijmegen, Holland), C. L. Meneghini (Bari, Italy), V. Pirilä (Helsinki, Finland), D. S. Wilkinson (High Wycombe, England)

and the

NORTH AMERICAN CONTACT DERMATITIS GROUP

Robert Adams, M.D., William E. Clendenning, M.D., Alexander A. Fisher, M.D., Norman Kanof, M.D., Walter G. Larsen, M.D., Howard Maibach, M.D., John C. Mitchell, M.D., Frances Storrs, M.D., Earl J. Rudner, M.D., William F. Schorr, M.D., James Taylor, M.D.

D0528500

MUNKSGAARD
COPENHAGEN

YEAR BOOK MEDICAL PUBLISHER
CHICAGO

Manual of Contact Dermatitis
2nd edition, 1st impression

Copyright © 1981 Munksgaard, Copenhagen

Printed in Denmark by P. J. Schmidt, Vojens

ISBN 87-16-08694-5

Distributed in North, South and Central America,
Hawaii and Puerto Rico by
Year Book Medical Publishers, Inc.

ISBN 0-8151-3282-4

Preface

The frequency of contact dermatitis is high among adults of both sexes, and dermatologists in their daily routine have many patients with this disease. To treat these patients properly, it is not enough to establish the diagnosis of contact dermatitis on morphological grounds. It is of the utmost importance to trace in each case the causes in the environment and the factors which are potential hazards. Numerous substances are involved and are present in many products and objects. It is necessary for dermatologists to have knowledge of chemical substances in both working and leisure time environments. Such substances and their presence in the environment are listed in this book.

It is not possible to cover all the sources of contact dermatitis because of the great local variation in industrialization, cosmetic habits and plant occurrence.

This book was planned as a manual for the dermatologist's routine work. The theoretical background of contact allergy is not included. For references and information necessary for more extensive investigation, the reader is referred to textbooks and monographs.

The book is written mainly for dermatologists who are not specialists in contact dermatitis. There is information of interest for industrial physicians, nurses, hygienists and safety engineers. The book may be used for postgraduate training in dermatology.

The second edition is revised according to new experiences, new publications and to helpful advice from readers.

I thank Professor Howard I. Maibach, San Francisco, for his invaluable assistance throughout the preparation of this book. He meticulously revised the style and grammar of the manuscript and offered many important suggestions and corrections to the contents.

Contents

1. Introduction and definition

Eczema or dermatitis is the name of a special inflammation in the skin; contact dermatitis refers to such an inflammation caused mainly by external agents. The names eczema and dermatitis are used for other inflammatory conditions of the skin not caused by external factors but mainly by endogenous factors. These include atopic dermatitis, seborrhoeic eczema, nummular eczema and stasis eczema. Not infrequently these conditions are complicated by the secondary development of contact dermatitis, for example from applied medicaments. Contact dermatitis (contact eczema) is divided into:

> Allergic contact dermatitis of delayed type
> Contact urticaria syndrom
> Irritant contact dermatitis of acute type
> Irritant contact dermatitis of chronic type
> Photoallergic contact dermatitis
> Phototoxic reaction

The frequency of contact dermatitis in a population is not known with certainty, but studies indicate that it amounts to several percentage points of the adult population. Contact dermatitis often accounts for 10 % or more of the patients admitted for skin diseases. The frequency can vary considerably from country to country and within one and the same country depending, among other things, on the degree of industrialization.

Often the disease is localized to the hands and can thus prevent the patient from working. Hand dermatitis in particular has a tendency to become "chronic" through repeated contacts. In some investigations, about 20 % of the cases of hand dermatitis were of occuptional origin.

If the contact dermatitis is treated properly, good results can be attained, even when the disease has lasted a long time. *Such treatment requires a detailed examination of the causes, which in turn demands a good knowledge of different occupations, hobbies, cosmetics and general environmental chemistry.*

Our chemical environment is incompletely explored as regards the damage it causes to the skin. *It is urgent to use the knowledge we already possess as well as we can.* In this book a general survey is given of the nature and cause of contact dermatitis, as well as some detailed information about the occurrence of the dermatitis-causing substances, and patch testing. In many cases, especially with regard to hand dermatitis occurring in gainful employment, a more detailed and comprehensive study is needed of, for example, the work place than has been described here.

2. The skin's defense against chemical and physical agents

The occurrence of contact dermatitis depends not only on external factors but also on the defensive powers on the skin, i. e. the ability to prevent penetration by dermatitis-causing agents and to neutralize such agents. The defensive powers vary considerably between individuals and between different parts of the skin on the same person.

The first line of defense is created by the *surface film* consisting of an emulsion of sebum, sweat and substances from the horny layer. Because it has acid character it has been called the skin's "acid mantle". Weak alkalis, considerably more harmful than weak acids, can be neutralized only to a slight extent. The film is probably not important in preventing penetration of substances; its main importance lies in its ability to prevent the horny layer from drying out. When the surface film is removed, e. g. by detergents and solvents, it usually takes hours to rebuild.

The principal line of defense lies in the *horny layer,* the stratum corneum, which among other things consists of keratin and "*water-binding substances*".

It is not known whether there are special cells or substances in epidermis or dermis which neutralize foreign chemicals.

It is the water content in the horny layer and not the fat content on the surface which is most important for the skin's "pliability". If the water-binding substances are produced in too small quantities or are removed by repeated use of detergents or solvents, dry skin with cracks is created.

In this way the possibilities for penetration are increased by dermatitis-causing substances. The water-binding substances can be replaced only on recreation of the horny layer, which takes days to weeks. It is important for dermatitis prophylaxis that they are not removed.

The dryness in the horny layer depends upon several factors, including the air humidity. If that is low, which is often the case indoors in the winter, the skin dries out and becomes "chapped". This is so especially when high air humidity suddenly drops to low while the barometric pressure simultaneously rises. The skin can then become dry in a few hours and remain chapped for several days.

Too great a skin humidity, e. g. through "wet" work, increases the skin's permeability. This is especially so if there is occlusion under, for example, rubber or plastic gloves, bracelets, rings, boots, tightly-fitting adhesive tape or in skin creases.

The horny layer's keratin can be damaged through the chemical chains being broken, especially by alkalis. In such injuries the underlying part of the epidermis is almost unprotected against external harmful factors.

3. Allergic contact dermatitis of delayed type

3.1 Contact allergy

(Cell mediated immunity, type IV hypersensitivity)

Contact allergy (contact sensitivity) involves an altered type of reaction in the skin, i.e. the allergy as such, does not cause a visible alteration. The skin can develop a dermatitis when it contacts those substances, the allergens, (=sensitizers) to which the allergy has been acquired. Allergic contact dermatitis is an inflammation which in its turn is a consequence of an immunological process. It contrasts with irritant reaction, where the inflammation is provoked by direct cell damage.

Hapten is the incomplete allergen which in skin is transferred into the complete allergen (antigen). In current usage hapten (e.g. formaldehyde, nickel-ion) is equal to allergen (sensitizer). Nearly all haptens have a molecular weight below 400 and rarely above 900. When a substance with higher molecular weight has given an allergic patch test reaction, a contaminant should be suspected.

Sensitization is the process of being sensitized. *Sensitivity* indicates that this process has occurred. *Sensitizing index* (or potential index) is the relative capacity of a given agent to induce sensitization in a group of human beings and animals.

Index of sensitivity is the incidence of acquired sensitivity to a given agent in a population compared with other agents.

Contact allergy is never inherited but is acquired after contact with certain substances. The origin of contact allergy, the sensitization, can occur after about a week's contact. Often it does not develop for years, sometimes decades.

The allergy is specific, i.e. in individual cases it involves one or a few definite substances.

Only a fairly small number of people normally acquire an allergy. Some few strongly allergenic substances can, however, give an allergy to most of the persons exposed, for example, poison ivy.

It cannot be predicted what people have a marked tendency to become sensitized.

Factors influenzing sensitization
Sensitization capacity of the chemical
Skin damaging factors
  Chemical, physical, skin disease, dryness, hydration
Environment
  Temperature, humidity, other chemicals
Exposure
  Concentration, occlusion, time, area
Genetic factors

There is no "safe" lower dose, even though industry representatives say so. It just takes longer to induce sensitization by a low dose.

The reaction can vary in intensity. In some cases a violent dermatitis is caused after a single contact, in other cases several hours' daily contact is needed. Percutaneous penetration of the substances plays a decisive part in the strength of the reaction and is determined by different characteristics in the substance, in the person and the skin area. In addition, the strength of the reaction depends upon the level of the allergy, which can vary even in the same person on different occasions.

To provoke a contact dermatitis once an allergy has been developed, often small quantities of the substances in question are required. Sometimes the quantity carried in the air, e. g. teak dust or turpentine vapor, is enough, or a brief touch of poison ivy. A dermatitis can most often be maintained by contact with such quantities of the substance as remain on a workbench or in pockets.

The allergy embraces the skin over the whole body. On renewed contact with the substance in question, the dermatitis is normally provoked at the place of the new contact, i. e. irrespective of where the contact occurred when the allergy began. Thus, for example, a sensitization to nickel can start through contact with nickel-plated

14

objects carried somewhere on the body, while the contact dermatitis later occurs on the hands through touching other nickel-plated objects.

The allergy normally remains for a long time, often for life. This is especially the case with substances with which we are in continual contact, e. g. nickel.

Once sensitization has taken place, a renewed contact of sufficient intensity gives rise to an allergic contact dermatitis. It sometimes happens that a patient is sensitized to several allergens present in different products (*simultaneous sensitivity*).

Cross sensitivity means that contact allergy caused by a *primary allergen* is combined with allergy to other chemically closely related substances, *secondary allergens*. This means that in those who have become sensitized to one substance, an allergic contact dermatitis, can be provoked or worsened by several other substances; this can apply even at the first contact with the latter. Cross sensitivity also exists between photoallergic substances.

Cross sensitivity should not be confused with the circumstance that the same substance can be present in several products (*false cross sensitivity*), e. g. in different balsams. Eugenol is present in numerous volatile oils, e. g. cinnamon, clove, allspice and bay leaf oil; these can then in turn form part of different products, e. g. perfumes, baked products and soft drinks.

Nor should cross sensitization be confused with the circumstance that certain sensitizers occur together in a product and that the sensitization to the different substances often then takes place on the same occasion (*concomitant sensitization*). Simultaneous sensitization occurs to nickel and cobalt on contact with nickel objects where cobalt is present as an impurity, and towards chromium and cobalt on contact with cement. The same applies to sensitizing to different rubber chemicals.

Examples of cross sensitizing groups are sulfonamides, organic color substances (p-phenylenediamine, azo-compounds), thiuram sulfides, certain antibiotics (neomycin, etc.) piperazine derivatives, hydrazines and catechols from different species of *Rhus,* sesquiterpene lactones in plants, parabens, phenothiazines, halogenated salicylanilides and nitrochlorobenzenes.

3.2 Clinical features

Provocation of allergic contact dermatitis in a previously sensitized person can occur after only one contact, e. g. from poison ivy, but usually it is a matter of repeated contacts, e. g. from rubber or nickel.

The allergic dermatitis is usually characterized by reddening, papules, vesicles, swelling and sometimes weeping and itching. Weeping suggests a strong allergic reaction or secondary infection.

When the dermatitis has been present for a while, the skin becomes dry and scaly and cannot be distinguished from an irritant dermatitis. Cracks often appear on the hands. Many factors affect the appearance such as the location of the dermatitis and the quantity of the allergen.

The nature of the allergen may decide the clinical appearance. Contact with plants can give streaklike erythema and bullae. Certain rubber chemicals (phenyl-isopropyl-p-phenylenediamine) can cause purpura-like dermatitis in industrial work and from boots. Film developer of p-phenylenediamine derivatives can cause lichen planus-like lesions. Zirconium (see Zirconium 4.8.6), mercury and beryllium can cause granulomatous dermatitis. Granulomas from stearate, silica, talc and magnesium are not of the allergic type. Pigmented dermatitis can be caused by perfumes in cosmetics.

In the sensitized person the allergic reaction causes skin lesions normally visible from 6-48 hours to several days after the contact.

"Chronic" allergic dermatitis is really prolonged acute dermatitis maintained by repeated allergen contact and irritants.

Dermatitis after one such contact can sometimes last for 1–2 weeks, that is why it is not necessary for more frequently renewed contacts to give a chronic appearance.

Nickel dermatitis has a tendency to spread to the arms and sometimes the body. Dermatitis on the lower legs from applied medicaments can spread suddenly over the remainder of the legs and thereafter generalize.

The initial localization is usually the most influential factor for the diagnosis; this can lead to special allergens being suspected.

About half of the contact dermatitis is located on the hands; of those which are occupational, about 90 % are on the hands. Irritant and allergic contact dermatitis is difficult to distinguish morphologically and often occurs at the same time. A primary allergic contact dermatitis is quickly complicated by an irritant dermatitis through irritants, e. g. detergents, easily penetrating the injured skin.

Usually allergic and irritant contact dermatitis is located dorsally. When the contact is caused by solid objects, e. g. nickel-plated objects, dermatitis of vesiculous type occurs in the palm. Allergic contact dermatitis from rubber tubes, handles, etc., can be located to the volar surface alone and characterized by redness and dryness without vesicles.

An irritant dermatitis can be complicated by a secondarily developed allergic contact dermatitis towards, e. g. rubber gloves or local treatment preparations. For obvious reasons, the hands are in contact with most known allergens.

The arms are often involved at the same time as the hands; sometimes the hands can be free if they have been protected by gloves or washed several times daily so that allergen contact has been minimal.

On the face allergic contact dermatitis is often localized around the eyes and swelling can occur. The allergens often can be transferred to the face via the hands even if the fingers are dermatitis free. Dust from teak or pollen from ragweed and gases can cause facial dermatitis. When an acute outbreak or chronic dermatitis occurs on the face, allergy to plants should be suspected, often from Compositae species. Work with unhardened epoxy products often causes hand and face dermatitis (see Photo contact dermatitis and Differential diagnosis).

Dermatitis on the lips caused by lipstick is usually characterized by dryness and scaling. The scalp seldom develops dermatitis. Hair dyes, etc., normally cause dermatitis away from the scalp (on the ears, forehead, eyelids and neck). Allergic contact dermatitis on eyelids may be caused by plants, eye makeup, face cream, nail polish or nickel via the fingers. Often the reaction on eyelids is of irritant, seborrhoeic or atopic type.

Dermatitis on the ear lobes is usually caused by earrings containing nickel.

Allergic dermatitis in the axillae is mainly from deodorants, antiperspirants and textiles.

Allergic contact dermatitis on the body is caused by dyes in clothes, elastics and nickel in buckles.

Dermatitis on legs and feet can be due to stockings, socks, boots and shoes. In stasis dermatitis or leg ulcers, secondary allergic dermatitis often occurs caused by the applied medicaments and bandages.

In the anal region, local treatment preparations of different types, e. g. local anesthetics for piles, are often responsible.

Dermatitis on the penis can be caused by condoms but is usually caused by substances transferred by the fingers without the latter necessarily having dermatitis.

Children below the age of 5 are sensitized less easily than adults. However, nickel dermatitis has been observed in the first year of life from zippers and buttons. Contact sensitivity to balsams seems common in children. Rhus dermatitis is common among American children. Rubber in toys and shoes can also sensitize.

Systemic symptoms such as nausea, diarrhea, fever and malaise occasionally may be present. These symptoms are probably due to intestinal allergic reactions. Sometimes patch testing can elicit the symptoms. Among such sensitizers are acrylates, sultones in alkylethersulfates, poison oak, pao ferro and teak.

3.3 Allergic reactions of mucous membranes

Contact reactions of the mucous membranes are rare. Reactions in the mouth show erythema and swelling; vesicles are uncommon. Dentures often have been blamed as causes of allergic reactions, but most reactions are of mechanical origin. Toothpastes, mouthwashes, dentures containing cobalt or nickel, anesthetics, antibiotics, impression pastes and surgical dressing (eugenol/colophony) and occasionally alcohol can cause allergic reactions in the mouth.

One reason why allergic reactions are rare might be that the saliva removes the sensitizers rather quickly. The subjective symptoms are often more pronounced than the objective ones. Stinging in the mouth and throat on exposure to dust or vapor is a stronger indication for irritant reaction than for allergic. Allergic reactions in the mouth are often accompanied by cheilitis: dryness and scaliness of the lips. Isolated angular cheilitis is often candidiasis. "Galvanism" in the mouth is a feeling of metal taste due to electric currents between different metals, e. g. mercury and gold, in fillings and dentures, and not a sign of allergic reaction.

The nasal mucosa can sometimes give reactions to nose drops containing antihistamines. In the conjunctiva, various drugs and preservatives in lens cleansers can cause allergic reactions. Allergic reactions on the vulva and vagina from perfumes in deodorants, chemical contraceptives, rubber pessaries and condoms are rare. Allergic reaction to copper in intrauterine devices is extremely rare.

4. The most common allergens (sensitizers)

4.1 Adhesives and tapes

(Cements, glues, pastes, plastic bonds, mucilages)

Gelatin and casein are of animal origin. Starch, dextrine, gum arabic, gum tragacanth, colophony (rosin), rubber latex, cellulose derivatives and shellac are of vegetable origin. Bitumen is a tar or oil product. Water-glass (sodium silicate) is an inorganic compound. Synthetic rubber and plastics used as adhesives are butyl latex, chloroprene (Neoprene), phenol-, carbamide- and melamine-formaldehyde, acrylic, polyvinyl acetate, alcohol and chloride, epoxy, saturated polyester (alkyd), unsaturated polyester, polystyrene, polyamide, coumarone-indene, polyurethane, thioplastics and organic silicones.

Sensitisers are colophony, formaldehyde resins, acrylic and epoxy resins, plasticizers (e. g. phthalates and tricresylphosfate), dyes, emulsifiers and preservatives such as formaldehyde, α-naphthol and chloracetamide. Thinners sometimes contain dipentene. The acrylic resin in tapes rarely sensitizes, but colophony and abitol (abietic alcohol) do. The sensitizing diphenyl thiourea can be used as a stabilizer in polyvinylchloride (PVC) tape.

4.2 Balsams, perfumes, flavoring agents and spices

Balsams are sweet-smelling mixtures of substances occurring in the plant kingdom. Every balsam contains several chemical compounds; many are identical in several balsams. Many contain both fragrance and flavor chemicals. Examples of balsams are balsam of Peru, tolu balsam, styrax, myrrh, galbanum, balsam of pine and spruce, colophony, gum benzoin, propolis (bee glue), and Karaya gum. This group includes the volatile oils in orange peel, citronella, cinnamon, cardamom, pepper, lavender, cloves (eugenol), neroli oil, pine needles, oil of laurel, vanilla, cajeput.

Contact with some balsams may occur directly in nature, e. g. pine and spruce, but the most common method of contact is via perfumes, spices and flavoring substances. Soft drinks may contain a number of balsams. Balsam of tolu is used as a tobacco fragrance.

Perfumes usually consist of a mixture of volatile oils. A change is being made from natural to synthetic scents, but the latter are also allergenic. Cinnamic aldehyde and alcohol, eugenol, isoeugenol, oak moss, hydroxycitronellal, geraniol, citronellol and jasmin are common perfume sensitizers. During "aging" of perfume the ingredients interact. That means that some substances lose the allergenicity and new sensitizers are formed. It is important to test with the actual batch. Athletes use larch turpentine on the hands and sportsmen use Tiger Balm® on skin for muscle pain. Balsam of Peru, eugenol and colophony are used in periodontal dressings. Karaya gum occurs in ostomy seal rings.

Perfumes are also present in floor and furniture polish, rubber, leather, drill oil, pesticides, detergents, soaps, etc. Probably more perfume is used in industrial products than in cosmetics. Since the presence of balsams is widespread in everyday life, it is often difficult to decide what product caused the dermatitis in a particular patient.

Balsam of Peru is usually used as a screening agent in patch testing; it detects about 50 % of the perfume allergies. Also mixtures of perfume substances are used for testing.

4.3 Clothing, shoes, personal objects

The most common substances in clothing causing dermatitis are dyes, rubber in elastics and nickel in buttons, hooks, buckles and zippers. There are other substances which generally are manufacturing secrets. Clothing dermatitis is not infrequently localized to the area around the axillae, where the sweat dissolves the substances. Rubber dermatitis occurs under bras and girdles. Nickel dermatitis is especially localized at the point of contact with the bra and with shoes, zipper fasteners, jeans buttons, etc.

Clothing dermatitis from formaldehyde resins has been recently less common. Green military uniforms may contain watersoluble tri-valent chromium, which can elicite dermatitis in chromium-sensitive persons.

In stockings it is often organic dyes that cause allergy. Black stockings (which need a large amount of dye) can provoke what is sometimes called a "mourning eczema". The dyes are generally related to p-phenylenediamine, azo- or antraquinonederivatives. The dermatitis is often localized to the popliteal fossa where sweating is greater and on the dorsal sides of the feet. Nonrubber fibers used in stretchable garments sometimes contain sensitizing mercaptobenzothiazole.

Gloves, especially when made of synthetic fibers, cause hand dermatitis. Usually the dye is responsible. Leather work gloves cause chromium allergy, especially in people with sweaty hands.

Shoes can cause allergic contact dermatitis from chromium in leather, dyes, rubber chemicals, nickel-plated accessories and antimildew agents. Glues in shoes commonly contain p-tert.-butylphenolformaldehyde resin. The sensitizing substances in vegetable tanning agents are usually not identified, but might be *Quebracho* extract and *Myrabolam* extract. Shoe leather dermatitis is often localized only to the dorsal side of the first toe.

Spectacle frames may contain sensitizers such as butylacrylate, tricresylphosphate and resorcinol monobenzoate (UV-absorber). Necklaces may be coated with incompletely cured epoxy resin. Sometimes they are made of exotic wood. Watchstraps may contain chromium compounds, organic dyes, phenol-formaldehyde resin.

4.4 Colophony (rosin)

Colophony is a resin obtained from pine and spruce trees. It contains abietic, hydroabietic and pimaric acids, coniferyl benzoate and several chemically undefined substances. Tall oil is a side product from the pulp industry. It contains fatty acids and up to 20 % resinous compounds (colophony). The potassium or trietanolamine soaps of tall oil fatty and resinous acids are used as emulsifiers in cutting oil, cleaning agents, rubber, etc. Abitol is the alcohol corresponding to hydroabietic acid. It is sticky and used in adhesive tapes and some cosmetics, e. g. mascara preparations. It does not cross-react to abietic acid.

Colophony is found in adhesive tape, felt tip pens, varnishes, insulating tape, labels, glossy paper, violin resin, some kitchen soaps and furniture polish. It is added to phenol-formaldehyde resin in glues and printing inks. Tall oil is used as an emulsifier in soluble cutting oils. Wrestlers gymnasts and squash players use it as an antislip substance on the hands. It has the same function on machine belts. Tin threads used in soldering contain colophony which evaporates when heated. It is used together with balsam of Peru and eugenol in periodontal dressings. In the wild we find it in pine and spruce wood.

It is often difficult to find the product responsible in an individual case with positive routine patch test reaction. When a tape is responsible, the dermatitis is often localized to the finger tips. Evaporated colophony from soldering tin threads may cause facial dermatitis.

4.5 Cosmetics and toiletries

Allergy to these preparations is fairly common, but when compared to the large number of consumers, this allergy is nevertheless uncommon. It should be pointed out that redness from cosmetics in, for example, face and axillae is not always of allergic but often of irritant type. Mascara preparations are often irritant.

The components which cause contact allergy are mainly perfumes (see Balsams 4.2), lanolin, preservatives, hair dyes (see Organic dyes 4.10) and colorants in eye shadow and lipsticks. Parabens, chloracetamide, chlorobenzene and chlorocresol derivatives, chloroxylenol and sorbic acid are used as preservatives.

Formaldehyde and formaldehyde releasers are used as preservatives in many cosmetics and are widely used in hair shampoos. They rarely sensitize in these low concentrations but can maintain hand dermatitis caused by, for example, formaldehyde plastics in low molecular form.

Among other sensitizers, mention may be made of resorcinol, isopropanol, chloro- and bromo-salicylanilides, hydroxyquinolines, probantheline bromide (antiperspirant). The antimicrobial agent 5-chloro-2-(2,4-dichloro-phenoxy)-phenol (Irgasan DP 300®) used in deodorants and toilet soaps is a rare sensitizer.

Sunscreening agents such as p-aminobenzoic acid (PABA) and its esters, and cinnamates can sensitize and more often photosensitize. Benzophenones, oxybenzone, dioxybenzone, anthranilates, digalloyl trioleate and benzylsalicylate rarely sensitize. It should be observed that there are cross-reactions between PABA esters and anesthetic agents of amine type.

Dermatitis from nail polish containing sulfonamide-formaldehyde or acrylic plastic is seldom localized to the area around the nails but rather to other sites via secondary contact from the nails, when it gives the appearance of streaky dermatitis on the skin or eyelid dermatitis. Artificial fingernails of methylmethacrylate or other acrylates can sensitize and cause paronychial reactions and onycholysis. Thioglycolates in permanent wave solutions are not allergens.

4.6 Formaldehyde

See also Plastics 4.15. Synonyms of formaldehyde: methanal, oxomethane, oxymethylene, methylene oxide, formic aldehyde, methyl aldehyde, formalith.

Formalin, a 37 % aqueous solution of formaldehyde, is present in certain plastics, preservatives, shampoos and dog shampoos, floor polish, certain detergents, glue, as a disinfectant, as a tanning agent in tanneries and as fixing agent for histological preparations, in water-resistant paper, wallboard. Textiles nowadays rarely release formaldehyde in amounts causing dermatitis.

Paraformaldehyde and hexamethylenetetramine gradually release formaldehyde. There are many other formaldehyde releasers on the market for glues, oils, paints, cosmetics, etc. Some sensitize without giving formaldehyde allergy. Patch testing with formaldehyde releasers in formaldehyde-sensitive individuals may give negative reaction due to the low continual release of formaldehyde.

If there is no contact with pure formaldehyde or glue, it can be difficult to determine from the case history what formaldehyde-containing product caused the dermatitis. Formaldehyde does not cross-react to glutaraldehyde, but this can be contaminated by formaldehyde.

Identification of formaldehyde
The sample (about 0.5-1 g of ointment, cream, oil, rubber, 3–5 cm² textile, etc.) is placed in a glass-stoppered glass jar (25–50 ml). In this jar is placed a glass tube (3–5 ml) containing 1 ml of chromatropic acid in conc. sulfuric acid (40 mg/10 ml). The jar is kept in darkness and the reaction read after 1 and 2 days. A violet color appears when formaldehyde is present. A red, brownish or yellowish color indicates presence of a chemical that disturbs the reaction. In this case it is not possible to detect formaldehyde by this method.

4.7 Medicaments

Contact allergy to drugs is more common than generally expected. If the medicament causes a strong local exacerbation of a dermatitis, the connection is easily made. Often, however, there is no such deterioration, especially if the skin disease is treated locally with corticosteroids at the same time. The symptoms can spread to the surrounding areas or other parts of the body, as the drug is transferred by the hands or the clothes. This is particularly common when the allergy has been caused by drugs used for leg eczema. Often the allergy can be completely concealed, especially when corticosteroid treatment is used. The only symptom in such a case may be the nonhealing of the original dermatosis.

These drugs sensitize not only the patients but also hospital personnel. Veterinarian medicaments can sensitize veterinarians and farmers.

Over the years the "offending" drugs have varied. Different periods have been dominated by mercury, sulfonamides, streptomycin, penicillin, neomycin and at present in certain countries ethylenediamine dihydrochloride in vehicles.

Antimicrobial agents are halogenated hydroxyquinolines, furacin, mercury compounds (thimerosal, phenyl-mercuric acetate, ammoniated mercury), xanthocillin, sulfonamides, resorcinol, chlorhexidine, chloracetamide, formaldehyde, acetarsol, and sorbic acid. Hexachlorophene rarely sensitizes, in spite of extensive use. Glutaraldehyde is used as sterilizing agent of instruments. It does not cross-react to formaldehyde, but may contain this compound.

Quaternary ammonium compounds are used as disinfectants, and may be present in solutions, creams, hand lotions, hair lotions, the gauze patch of adhesive tape for wounds, eye and ear drops. It is used in antistatic cleansers. Sensitization does occur but is rare. The test reactions of irritant type might be misinterpreted as allergic. The anti-viral agent Idoxuridine (5-I-2-deoxy-uridine) for treatment of herpes simplex and tromantadine-HCl can sensitize.

Among antibiotics, the partly cross-reacting drugs neomycin, gentamycin, tobramycin, kanamycin are the most common. Framycetin contains $> 99\%$ of neomycin B and $< 1\%$ of neomycin C. Chloramphenicol, tetracycline derivatives, virginiamycin and polymyxin B can sensitize. Erythromycin base can sensitize but the stearate seems to be safe. Penicillin of different types can sometimes sensitize pharmaceutical, veterinarian and hospital personnel.

Most antimycotic preparations can sensitize. To this group belong dichlorophene, hydroxyquinolines, tolnaftate and chlorosalicylamide (photosensitizer), p-hydroxybenzoates (parabens), sulbetine, clotrimazole, buclosamide (photosensitizer), miconazole nitrate 3-ethylamino-1, 2-benzisothiazol-HCl, pyrrolnitril, dihydroxy-dichloro-diphenyl-sulfide and -methane. Antimycotics are sometimes used as preservatives in deodorants. Undecylenic acid is not an allergen and may be used as a substitute.

Many antihistamines sensitize, and should be avoided as local treatment of dermatitis.

The antiinflammatory agents phenylbutazone and oxyphenbutazone sometimes sensitize when applied locally.

26

Agents for depigmentation, e. g. monobenzylether of hydroquinone and hydroquinone sometimes sensitize, but are more usually irritants.

Balsams, e. g. of Peru, occur in some wound dressings and suppositories. Colophony, eugenol and balsam of Peru are used in periodontal dressing. Sensitizing Karaya gum may occur in the appliance adhesive around stoma.

Local anesthetic preparations derivatived from p-aminobenzoic acid, e. g. benzocaine, procaine, tetracaine, butacaine, can mutually cross-sensitize. Benzocaine often occurs in preparations for wounds and burns in homes and industry. Lidocaine (Lignocaine, Xylocaine), mepivacaine (carbocaine), bupivacaine and prilocaine rarely sensitize.

Corticosteroids can sensitize, particularly in patients with leg dermatitis and external otitis. Also oral, intralesional and intra-articular application can induce sensitization. They do not cross-react.

Tars (wood, coal) infrequently sensitize. Phototoxic reactions are seen. Those who become allergic to wood tars are often also allergic to rosin, perfumes and balsam of Peru.

Other medicaments such as vitamin A (retinoic acid), epinephrine, nitrogen mustard, fluorouracil and nitroglycerin ointment sensitize.

Ointment bases have a sensitizing capacity, especially lanolin and the stabilizing agent ethylendiamine-dihydrochloride. Ethylene and propylene glycol can sensitize. Yellow and white petrolatum (Vaseline®) are so rarely sensitizing that they are used as bases in patch testing. The allergen is unknown.

Sensitizing preservatives in the ointment/cream bases, in eye drops and cleansing liquids for eye contact lenses are particularly p-hydroxy-benzoic acid derivatives (parabens), p-chloro-m-cresol, p-chloro-m-xylenol (PCMX), and organic mercury compounds. Ethylenediamine tetraacetate (EDTA) used in eye drops does not sensitize or cross-react to ethylenediamine.

Adhesive tape (see 4.1) contains colophony and antioxidants. Wound dressings may contain quaternary ammonium compounds.

4.8 Metals

4.8.1 Chromium

Hexavalent chromium (chromate and bichromate) and trivalent chromium are allergenic. Hexavalent chromium penetrates more easily into the skin and is of greater importance as a cause of dermatitis. Probably hexavalent chromium is reduced into trivalent in the skin when as a hapten it conjugates to form the antigen. Chromium metal and stainless steel do not yield chromium in a soluble form if not affected by certain chemicals and so do not sensitize.

Chromium valences

Cr^0
* metal in alloys (e. g. stainless steel) and in plating not soluble, not sensitizing

Cr^{3+}
* salts of inorganic acids (e. g. chlorides), soluble, sensitizing, may precipitate in alkaline environment
* salts of organic acids (e. g. oxalate), soluble, sensitizing
* basic sulfate (leather tanning agent), soluble, sensitizing
* oxide (Cr_2O_3), not soluble, not sensitizing
* hydroxides, when aged not soluble, and then not sensitizing
* complexes used in textile dyes, commonly not sensitizing

Cr^{4+}
* dioxide (in magnetic tapes) forms Cr^{6+} and Cr^{3+} in presence of water, sensitizing

Cr^{6+}
* chromates, dichromates of K-,Na-,Ca-,NH_4-,dichromate of Zn, soluble, sensitizing
* chromate of Zn, chromate and dichromate of Pb, weakly soluble, weakly sensitizing

The most common cause of chromium dermatitis is *cement*. Bricklayers, cement workers and layers of paving stones are often affected. The cement dermatitis on the dorsal side of the hands has often a patchy feature. The chromate derives mainly from the raw material which contains trivalent chromium like all earth crust material. It is partly oxidized to hexavalent form in the cement kiln. Water soluble chromate (the sensitizing part) occurs commonly up to 15 μg Cr/g, sometimes up to 50 μg. The water soluble amount is not correlated to the total amount.

In wood ash there is chromate to an equally high concentration as in cement; it can maintain a hand dermatitis. Other common chromate contacts are plating baths, bichromate sulfuric acid for cleaning of laboratory glass, chromic acid for rust protection, chromium compounds in offset printing, green uniforms, and green baize on gaming tables. Liberated chromate in welding fumes causes dermatitis on the face. This is particularly the case when stainless steel is welded as the rod contains chromium metal, which might be oxidized and the coating of these electrodes contains chromate. When these electrodes are manufactured, the wet coating may sensitize.

Antirust paints contain besides the barely soluble lead, zinc and barium chromates, also soluble alkali chromates, causing these products to sensitize. Common chromate paints (yellow/red) do not contain alkali chromates, so they rarely sensitize. Barely soluble chromates are used as pigments in rubber and printing ink.

Soluble cutting oil used for swarfing, etc., dissolves chromate applied as antirust paint on iron. Zinc galvanized iron sheets are coated by chromium compounds, partly water soluble six valent, to prevent the formation of "white stain". Chromate can easily contaminate the hands in mg amounts. When ventilation pipes are made from these sheets in machines, the rolling oil used is contaminated by chromate and can be transferred to skin. Certain types of magnetic tapes for sound or television contain chromium dioxide. When in contact with water, for example on the fingers, some part of the chromium dioxide is transformed into water soluble chromate. Sensitization is rare as small amounts are released. Brickstones used as lining in refractory furnaces contain a large amount of trivalent chromium. This can be oxidized into hexavalent form by heat in alkaline environment. The ash or lining material at kiln repair can then sensitize. Chromate is often used as a preservative in milk samples for estimation of lipid and protein content. Chromate may be used in the curing process of polyvinyl alcohol and certain acrylates.

Chromium dermatitis often has a chronic character as hidden sources of chromium compounds are present in the daily environment. Among these are matches. Fragments from the match head can soil the pockets. When the match head is touched, chromate is transferred to the hands (especially if they are sweaty or wet). When ashtrays are washed or cleaned, contact takes place easily with chromate-containing burnt match heads which can cause dermatitis in people doing household work and cleaning. Common detergents do not contain chromium compounds in any amount or form that causes allergic contact dermatitis. Eau de Javelle contains chromate in some countries.

Trivalent complex chromium compounds (basic chromium sulfate) used as leather tanning agents penetrate skin and cause dermatitis in tanners. After the leather has been affected for a while by sweat, the chromium linkage to leather collagen is broken, whereupon it can come into contact with skin from work gloves and shoes. Dog leashes may be made of leather and release sensitizing chromium compound on sweaty hands; a leather purse in a trouserpocket can cause thigh dermatitis. Trivalent chromium in green tattoos can induce sensitization and local dermatitis after several years.

Photopatch testing results indicate increased light sensitivity in patients with chromate dermatitis.

4.8.2 Nickel

As opposed to chromium, nickel metal is allergenic as it is dissolved on the skin surface. In fact it is the major cause of nickel dermatitis. It occurs generally as nickel plating, i. e. as nickel on the surface of another metal and in several alloys, e.g. coins. Stainless steel contains nickel, but so firmly bound that it is not released if not affected by certain chemicals. Nickel salts can cause dermatitis; this is particularly common in nickel plating. Nickel oxides are allergens and occur in green pigment, which forms part of paint and glass or ceramic enamel.

Many objects, e. g. water taps and spectacles have nickel plating under the chromium plating. This emerges after a few years' wear. Nickel is also often present under gold plating of jewelry. Gold and rodium plated spectacles are nickel plated underneath. Gold and rodium are eroded by sweat. Silver and 'white gold" jewelry often contains 10 % nickel. "Silver" threads in electronics often contain more than 50 % nickel. Nickel in alloys can be released into soluble cutting oil.

Contact occurs at work, but also in objects such as shoes, press studs, hooks, zippers, buckles, jewelry, cigarette lighters, pens, purse locks, lipstick holders, powder compacts, wristwatch buckles, hairpins, keys, coins, pen knives, drawer handles and scissors. Nowadays buttons in jeans often cause sensitization in both sexes and elicite dermatitis on the abdomen. Detergents do not contain nickel in any amount or form that causes allergic contact dermatitis.

In women, nickel dermatitis often starts under personal apparel Data on such dermatitis may sometimes be found in case histories going back many years. Patients then change to objects of plastic or other metals. About 10 % of women in the normal population are sensitive to nickel. The allergy persists, and if the hands are exposed to irritant factors, e. g. continuous cleaning, they become so damaged that nickel enters the skin more easily and a hand dermatitis arises. Once the hand nickel dermatitis has started it is difficult to heal.

Nickel dermatitis has a certain tendency to spread over the arms and the rest of the body. Sometimes this results from the nickel being transferred via the fingers. Less frequently, a spreading of the dermatitis takes place after surgery, when nickel is absorbed in the operation scar.

Nickel in food can probably aggravate and cause chronicity of dermatitis on the hands. It is not possible to give reliable advice on a nickel-deficient diet as the content of nickel in food, particularly vegetables and fruit, is influenced by several factors. Sour vegetables and salt can release nickel from cooking utensiles of stainless steel. Cacao and tea contain a relatively high amount.

Spot test for detection of nickel: A few drops of 1 % dimethyl-glyoxime in ethanol solution and 10 % ammonium hydroxide solution are successively applied on a cotton-tipped applicator. The tip is rubbed against the metal object. A strawberry red color on the cotton indicates the presence of nickel. The solutions can be applied as a spot test on the object or added to solutions. Patients can perform this test at home and at work.

4.8.3 Cobalt

Cobalt metal is allergenic like nickel metal to which it is closely related. Cobalt exists in daily life mainly as an impurity in nickel metal. Cement is the most common cause of cobalt allergy in the working environment. Of those who have cement dermatitis and have been sensitized to chromium, one-third have been sensitized to cobalt.

Allergenic oxides of cobalt occur in pigment used for painting of pictures and china and in enamelling. The dried paint or the baked enamel is not an allergen thanks to its insolubility. Blue tattoo markings may contain cobalt oxide. As a drying agent cobalt occurs in linseed oil and certain printing inks. It is also used in cold cured acrylics and unsaturated polyester plastic but then rarely sensitizes. Hard metal alloys can release cobalt into soluble cutting oils. Dentures can release cobalt and give allergic reactions in the mucosa. Certain types of magnetic tapes for sound and television contain small amounts of cobalt, but sensitization is rare. Cobalt salts are used as humidity registration agents. Cobalt is used as a catalyst in butadiene rubber.

Isolated cobalt contact allergy found by routine testing, particularly in women, is often not explainable.

4.8.4 Chromium/nickel/cobalt

There is often allergy against two or three of the metals at the same time in different combinations. The presence of chromium and cobalt in cement means that this combination is most common in men. On the other hand, the simultaneous presence of nickel and cobalt in nickel-plated objects means that women display more of this combined allergy against nickel and cobalt. *The chromium allergy as such is one of the most common allergies in men, while nickel allergy is one of the most common among women.*

4.8.5 Metallic implants

Tissue fluids may produce corrosion of metallic foreign bodies, e. g. hip prostheses, valve replacements, bone screws or ligatures, pacemaker electrodes, intravenous cannulae, dental nails. Metal-to-metal hip prostheses are more corroded than metal-to-plastic, but they are now less used than previously. Released cobalt and nickel rarely induce contact allergy. Some cases with contact allergy to these metals acquired before the implantation may develop local inflammation or/and exacerbation of dermatitis. In patients allergic to cobalt, the alloy Vitallium should not be used as it contains about 60% cobalt, but Charnley should be used instead. Local inflammation in hip prostheses is often caused by anaerobic infection. Osteomyelitis from metal osteosynthesis in a nickel-sensitive person has been reported. Patients may have metal allergy without rejection of the hip prostheses. Pacemakers are made of titanium which is insoluble in body fluids and does not cause allergic reaction. (Previously pacemakers were epoxy resin coated).

Loosening of hip prosthesis may also be due to plastic components such as methylmethacrylate or benzoylperoxide.

4.8.6 Other metals

Mercury allergy was previously more common than it is now. The reason is probably a reduced or discontinued use of sublimate and ammoniated mercury as applied medicaments and disinfectants.

The metal is, like nickel and cobalt, allergenic. It can cause allergic dermatitis at the manufacturing of instruments or the preparation of amalgam for dental fillings (the hardened amalgam in the mouth does not sensitize). Mercury metal may occur in antifreckle creams. Mercury metal which has penetrated down into the skin can cause granuloma. Red mercury sulfide is used in artists' paints and in tattoos. The dermatitis may appear many years after tattooing.

Organic mercury compounds sometimes sensitize when they are used as tanner's mordant or preservatives in drugs. Among these compounds is merthiolate (thimerosal, thiomersalate, sodium ethylmercurithiosalicylate).

Gold metal in jewelry and dentures and gold salts in plating solutions rarely sensitize.

Platinum salts are strong sensitizers, but the metal is not (see Contact urticaria, 6).

Zirconium sodium lactate sometimes gave allergic granulomas when used in antiperspirants; it is now replaced by zirconyl hydroxychloride which does not sensitize. Zirconium oxide used for treatment of Rhus plant dermatitis can cause allergic granulomas.

Copper salts and metal rarely sensitize.

Lead salts and metal affected by acids rarely sensitize. Lead cyanamide in antirust may sensitize.

Iodine is now a rare sensitizer.

Beryllium, a strong sensitizer, rarely produces dermatitis since it has a limited use in special alloys. It can cause granuloma.

Antimony and arsenic compounds have been reported as sensitizers, but the findings are controversial.

Phosphorus sesquisulfide present in "strike-anywhere" matches and in "lightning paper" sometimes causes allergic contact dermatitis.

Iron, zinc and cadmium fortunately do not cause contact allergic dermatitis.

4.9 Oils and petrols

There are many different kinds of industrial oils: casting, grinding, drilling, cutting, lubricating, moulding, hydraulic, rolling, hardening, and impregnation oils. There are many brands and labeling of the ingredients is often incomplete.

The bases consist of petroleum products, vegetable oils, animal fatty acids, synthetic compounds (polyglycols, polyglycolethers, etc.). The oils can be sulfated and chlorinated and are then more irritant. Many additives are employed. Most cutting oils are emulsions, requiring antimicrobial agents such as chloracetamide, formaldehyde releasers, Grotan BK (a triazine), N-methylol-chloracetamide, p-chloro-m-cresol, 1,2-benzisothiazoline-3-one, salicylanilides. Antioxidants (e. g. phenolic derivatives), rust preventives, ethylenediamine, acrylates, p-phenylenediamine, derivatives, azo dyes, perfumes (e. g. pine oil), hydrazine, chromate, dichlorophene, mercaptobenzthiazole are among the known sensitizers. Tall oil containing sensitizing colophony is often used as an emulsifier. Also soaps made of tall oil (see 4.4) used as cutting oil may cause sensitization to colophony.

Soluble cutting oil may be contaminated by chromate from

painted metal and by nickel and cobalt from metal pieces and tools. Between 20 and 50 % of oil dermatitis cases have been considered to be of allergic type.

An irritant reaction is easily provoked on testing with oil. If the oil is diluted instead, the concentration of the added substances becomes low yielding a false negative reaction as a consequence. For this reason, many cases of allergic dermatitis which occur in work with oil are probably overlooked and interpreted as irritant contact dermatitis.

Several dyes, also of azo type, are added to petrol (gasoline).

4.10 Organic dyes

Organic dyes exist in several different types; those which sensitize most are derivatives of aniline, p-phenylenediamine, azobenzene and benzidine. Several tend to cross-react at testing. Dyes of antraquinone, nigrosin and pyrazolon are often less sensitizing. Rosaniline, malachite green, brilliant green and crystal violet are examples of triphenyl methane dyes which sensitize less frequently. Eosin, earlier used especially for lipsticks, can photosensitize, but it is not used at present.

The different dyes can occur in textiles, furs, leather, hair dyes, hair tints, ballpoint pens, plastics, cosmetics, household and sanitary paper, food and drugs. Dyes added to petrol (gasoline) to differentiate between octane numbers are of azo-type.

The most common hair dyes are p-phenylenediamine, p-toluenediamine, p-aminodiphenylamine, 2,4-diaminoanisol, o-aminophenol. Different colors are obtained by couplers such as resorcinol, hydroquinone, catechol, naphthol, 2,5-xylenol and m-phenylenediamine. p-Toluene diamine has replaced p-phenylenediamine in several countries as a hair dye and is claimed to be less sensitizing, but we have no evidence of this.

p-Phenylenediamine derivatives used as antioxidants in rubber and oils do not cross-sensitize to p-phenylenediamine. 4,4-Diaminodiphenylmethane used in epoxy systems, polyurethanes and in rubber cross-reacts as do several dyes of azo-type.

The chemistry of many dyes can be identified from their color index number (C.I. No.) (see References). More than 1,000 dyes are used in the textile industry.

4.11 Paints

Paints contain bases, solvents, pigments and additives. Hardeners are added to some paints when used.

The bases are mostly synthetic polymers which do not sensitize, e. g. alkyd (saturated polyester), polyvinyl chloride, -acetate, -butyral, acrylates, polyurethanes. Other bases contain monomers which might be sensitizers, e.g. epoxy-, phenol/formaldehyde-, urea/ formaldehyde-melamin/formaldehyde-, urethane-resins. Hardeners may sensitize (see Plastics 4.15). The bases may contain natural products, e. g. colophony. Linseed oil paints are now rare. They contained cobalt products as dryers and turpentine as an oxidizing agent.

The common solvents are petroleum products (White spirit, kerosene, etc.) which are nonsensitizers. Turpentine is rarely used but dipentene (limonene) may be present in thinners. Plasticizers and other additives rarely sensitize. Because of the risk of neurotoxic effect of solvents, water-based paints are widely used. Emulsifiers make it possible to decrease the amount of solvent and to add water instead. Then preservatives often are necessary; these can sensitize e. g. chloracetamide (see Preservatives 4.16).

Among pigments, chromate might sensitize but rarely because the solubility of the used chromates is low (see Chromium 4.8.1). Cobalt oxides are still used in artists' paints but commonly not in industrial paints. Other pigments or dyes in paints rarely sensitize.

4.12 Pesticides

The range of pesticides is large; several can cause allergic dermatitis.

The thiuramsulfides (TMTD, TMTM etc.) and dithiocarbamates (Ziram, Ferbam, Maneb, Zineb, Nabam, etc.) are well-known sensitizers also when used in rubber. Thiuramsulfides are decomposed to dithiocarbamates and these to thiourea.

Thiuramsulfides and dithiocarbamates are often used on roses in gardens. Other pesticides reported as sensitizers are captan, ethylenediamine, mercaptobenzothiazole, rodannitrobenzene, dithianone, dichlorvos, o-difolatan, atrazine, benomyl, o-o-dietyl-phtalimido-phosphothioate, nitrofurazone, naphthylthiourea, 2,6-dinitro-o-cresol, diethyl-phthalimido-phosphothioate, captafol. Pyrethrum is produced from a chrysanthemum species. It is present in insecticides, but is then purified and nonsensitizing.

4.13. Photographic chemicals

For developing black and white film, metol (methylaminophenol sulfate) and TSS (4-amino-N,N′-diethylaniline) are used, while several chemicals are needed for developing color film. Most are derivatives of p-phenylenediamine or aniline, e. g. CD-2 (3-methyl-4-amino-N-diethylaniline-HCl) and CD-3 (2-amino-5-diethyl-aminotoluene-HCl). Color film developers and TSS can cause a lichen planus-like eruption. Fixing agents normally do not provoke contact allergy

For photocopying, several chemicals are used, some of which are related to p-phenylenediamine, which is also part of both organic dyes and rubber chemicals. p-tert. Butylcatechol and resorcinol are sometimes used and are sensitizing. Dimethylthiourea is used in azo papers and is both a sensitizer and photosensitizer.

4.14 Plants and woods

Acute and chronic dermatitis on the face should always be suspected to be caused by plants. Particularly Compositae and lichen dermatitis can simulate atopic or phytophoto dermatitis. Erythema multiformelike symptoms may occur in pao ferro-sensitized individuals.

Patch tests should be performed with the plants recognized as causing the actual dermatitis, as the content of allergen can vary among specimens. Different parts of the plants should be used.

Many plants are irritants and controls have to be tested. Wood dust should be dry, used as is and 10% in petrolatum. As far as possible the species of wood or plant should be determined.

Plants and wood can occur as special products such as wood dust, perfume, rosin, spices, turpentine, beverages, food, cosmetics, and popular topical medicaments such as Arnica tincture and Camomille extract.

Compositae family, particularly *Chrysanthemum,* contains most allergenic species. They contain about 600 sesquiterpene lactones; many cross-react. Some species cross-react with *Frullania* (liverworth) and some lichens.

Rhus (poison ivy, oak and sumac) causes not only most cases of plant dermatitis in the US but probably also most cases of allergic contact dermatitis. In some areas these plants are a common cause of occupational dermatitis. Pentadecylcatechol in poison ivy is a strong sensitizer, but different catechols present cross-react. *Rhus* belongs to the Anacardiaceae family, like the cashew nut tree and mango; more than 20 genera are allergenic. The contact usually takes place by direct touch but may occur via contaminated tools or clothing.

Ragweed (ambrosia) produces contact dermatitis through its content of an oil soluble oleoresin. (Asthma and rhinitis are caused by a water soluble substance). The face is often affected and the dermatitis can simulate photo contact dermatitis.

Other important sensitizing plants are philodendron and oleander. Lilies, tulips, narcissus, alstromeria and daffodils cause allergic contact dermatitis through bulbs and other parts of plants.

In Europe *Primula obconica* is one of the most common causes of plant dermatitis. It is also found in the US.

Certain lichens and the liverwort *Frullania* which grow on trees cause "woodcutter's eczema". Lichens also grow on stones and cement walls.

Some vegetables can sensitize, e. g. lettuce. Allergic contact dermatitis from vegetables, onion and garlic in chefs is often located to fingertips of the three radial fingers of the left hand.

Tobacco itself rarely sensitizes, but pipe tobacco can cause finger dermatitis by its content of Balsam of tolu or other fragrances.

More than 100 species of trees are known to contain sensitizers. Contact usually occurs on sawing and polishing. The trade names are often misleading. One species can have several trade names and different species can have the same trade name. Some common ones are *Khaya anthoteca* (khaya), *Tectona grandis* (teak), *Dalbergia latifolia* (Jacaranda = Rio palisander), *Chlorophora excelsia* (Iroko = kambala), *Macherium scleroxylon* (Pao ferro), *Swientenia macrophylla* (Mahogany), ebony, cedar.

The frequency of plant dermatitis varies among different parts of the world, e. g. *Radiata pine* and bush dermatitis in Australia, *Parthenium hysterophorus* dermatitis in India, *Rhus* dermatitis in USA and *Primula obconica* dermatitis in Europe.

The chemical formula for certain plant sensitizers is known: Poison ivy (pentadecylcatechol and other catechols), *Primula obconica* (primin), tulip and *alstromeria* (α-methylene-γ-butyrolactone), some species of *chrysanthemum* (sesquiterpene lactones), *Frullania* (sesquiterpene lactones), some species of teak (dimethoxydalbergion, anthotecol, etc.), ragweed oleoresin (sesquiterpene lactones), iroko (chlorophorin), *Tectona grandis* (lapachol). Sensitizers in lichens are atranorin, evernic acid, usnic acid, sesquiterpene lactones and several others. Owing to chemical relationships between quinones, cross-reactions occur between teak, palisander and *Primula obconica*. Pine and spruce balsams often show simultaneous patch test reactions to balsam of Peru, colophony and wood tar.

See also "Balsam", "Turpentine", "Irritants", "Phototoxic contact dermatitis" and "Contact urticaria".

4.15 Plastics

Plastics consist of large molecules which are not in general allergenic. Exceptions to this are especially formaldehyde plastics which give off formaldehyde. The allergic dermatitis occurs when work is done with semicured products (resins, hardeners or other substances). Sometimes the cured products contain leachable additives causing contact allergy

Formaldehyde resins

The formaldehyde resins usually consist of formaldehyde linked to carbamide (urea), melamine or phenols. The formaldehyde itself and the low molecular compounds can be allergens. Carbamide resin and melamine resin are usually colorless and phenol resin (bakelite) is black or brown. Carbamide- and melamine resins together are named aminoplastics.

Carbamide resin is used for making textiles crease-free, gluing of wood, permanent treatment of parquet flooring, in paints, etc. Playing cards are usually covered with carbamide resin. It improves water resistance of paper and household paper. When the resin occurs in textiles, the dermatitis is usually localized to exposed parts of the body. Such dermatitis is now rare. It normally causes hand dermatitis when worked in semicondensed form. p-Toluene sulfonic acid used as hardener is a rare sensitizer.

Melamine resin is often found on the surface of laminated tables, benches and walls.

Phenol resin is used for the production of bakelite products and for the gluing of wood, leather (shoes, watchstraps), rubber and metal. p-tert. Butylphenol-resin may occur to excess and cause contact allergy (as wall as leucoderma). Phenol resin is mixed with sand for iron casting. Some resins are used as epoxy hardeners.

Contact allergy to carbamide and melamine resin is normally combined with formaldehyde allergy. This is not so with phenol resin, which in low molecular form is allergenic. Many different phenols are used (phenol, cresol, resorcinol, p-tert. butylphenol, etc.) and the manufacturing processes vary. The different resins (resols, novolacks, etc.) do not cross-react; patch tests should be performed with actual products besides the common, for example, that of p-tert. butylphenol. Some contain surplus hexamethylenetetramine; the sensitivity is not always combined with formaldehyde allergy. One of the allergens in p.tert.-buthylphenol formaldehyde resin is 2-hydroxy-5-tert.-butyl-benzylalcohol.

Epoxy resin

Most industrial epoxy resins are of the bisphenol A type. The low molecular oligomer (MW, molecular weight 340) is the main sensitizer. "Low molecular" resins are mixtures of low molecular oligomers, mainly MW 340, with an average MW below 1000. "High molecular" resins are mixtures of high molecular oligomers with an average MW above 1000, but there are traces of MW 340 oligomer.

Mainly low molecular epoxy resin sensitizes. High molecular epoxy resin dissolved in solvents for painting or epoxy resin powder for electrostatic coating of metal rarely causes sensitization owing to the low content of oligomer MW 340. However, dermatitis might be elicited in previously sensitized individuals.

This resin is used extensively because of its extraordinary technical qualities. Of the new products in industry, the epoxy resin system is one of the most common causes of allergic contact dermatitis. Sensitization may occur after only a few contacts. The dermatitis is localized to the hands but often also to the face.

The allergy may be caused not only by the oligomers but also by the hardeners (curing agents) and reactive diluents. Most *hardeners* used in thermal hardening seem harmless, e.g. phthalic anhydride and dicyandiamide.

The most potent sensitizers among the hardeners are the aliphatic amines, e. g. ethylenediamine (also present in certain ointments), diethylenetriamine (DETA), triethylenetetramine (TETA), dipropylenetriamine, dimethylaminopropylamine, tetraethylenepentamine, isophorondiamine, trimethylhexamethylenediamine and 4,4-diamino-diphenylmethane and piperazine derivatives. Hardeners of the polyamide type are much safer (but may contain traces of sensitizing aliphatic amine) as are anhydrides. Sensitizing phenol-formaldehyde resins are used as hardeners. Several hardeners of adduct type (e. g. epoxy resin/aliphatic amine) are weak sensitizers or not sensitizers at all.

The reactive diluents such as butyl-cresyl- and phenylglycidylether are strong sensitizers. The long chain aliphatic Epoxide 8 is a sensitizer.

Up to 25 % of the resin can remain unhardened, particularly when cured at room temperature. This unhardened resin rarely induces sensitization but can elicite dermatitis in sensitive individuals and cause "chronic" dermatitis. Preimpregnated glassfibers ("prepreg") used as reinforcement in plastic industry and in electronic circuit sheets are only partly hardened and can sensitize.

Epoxy resin is used for the casting of models, engine covers, electric insulation, connecting of cables, floor covering, paint for chemical-resistant floors and walls, anticorrosion protection of metals, waterproof concrete, mending of cracks in concrete and as glue for metal, plastic, rubber and ceramics. Commercially it is available as glue for "do-it-yourself". It is also used by dentists for fillings. Epoxy products are commonly marketed as "two-component" systems.

For electronics and electron microscopy, other types are often used and the sensitizing nonenyl- and dodecenyl-succinic anhydride may be used as hardeners.

Acrylates

Acrylic plastic of methylmethacrylate is in itself clear and is used in plexiglass. Dermatitis from this acrylate occurs mainly in dental technicians who make and mend dentures. It is the monomer which is allergenic and only exceptionally the finished product contains unhardened traces. Oral lesions are often believed to be due to denture allergy but it is nearly always a pressure effect. Testing of scrapings from the denture is rarely positive but methylmethacrylate must be used. Acrylic plastic is used for locking screws/nuts, hearing aid apparatus, floorlaying, tightening, in leather finishing, adhesives, paints, oil additives, artificial rubber and histological preparations. When used in orthopedic surgery, it can penetrate rubber gloves and cause hand dermatitis.

Acrylates (methyl-, ethyl-, butyl-, ethylhexyl-, hydroxybutyl-, etc.) are extensively used by industry. The low molecular acrylates in glues may sensitize but not the high molecular ones in paint and textile and rarely when in adhesive tape. In some acrylates sensitizing additives are present, e.g. dimethyl-p-toluidine, hydroquinone, pyrogallol, resorcinol. When dentures and synthetic joints are made, liquid acrylic monomer is mixed with methylmethacrylate powder containing the sensitizing catalyst benzoylperoxide. Sometimes hydroxyethylmethacrylate is added to the liquid monomer.

Acrylic compounds hardened by UV-light are now widely used.

They contain several sensitizers: prepolymers, e.g. acrylated polyesters, acrylated epoxy resin and multifunctional acrylic esters, e. g. pentaerythritol triacrylate (PETA). These compounds contain two or more vinyl groups ($CH_2 = CH-$) which are allergenic. Products may contain photoinitiators (benzophenone derivatives, dimethylaniline, benzoin, etc.), monoacrylates (2-ethylhexylacrylate, etc.), inhibitors (phenthiazines, hydroquinone, hydroquinone monobenzylether), accelerators (amines, mercaptocompounds, phosphine derivatives), stabilizers (thiuram sulfides), pigments, dyes, formaldehyde resin. These products are used in printing ink, printing plates, metal varnish, textile finish, electronics and dentistry. The prepolymers and multifunctional acrylic esters are not allergenic after hardening.

Polyurethanes
These plastics are made from polyols and isocyanates. The polyols are not sensitizers. 4,4′-Diisocyanate dicyclohexyl methane, diphenylmethane-4,4-diisocyanate (MDI), polymethylene-polyphenylisocyanate (PAPI), 3-isocyanate-methyl-3,5,5-trimethyl-cyclohexylisocyanate (IPDI) and hexamethylene-1,6-diisocyanate (HMDI) sometimes sensitize. Toluene-diisocyanates (2,4-TDI and 2,6-TDI) do not sensitize. Diaminodiphenylmethane (methylenedianiline, dianilinomethane) (DDM) and isophoronediamine (IPD) are sensitizers, which also occur in epoxy systems. DDM occurs in rubber.

Polyester plastics
Unsaturated polyester plastic mixed with styrene reinforced with glass fiber is a strong material from which tubes, transparent roofing, etc., are made. It is used for gluing of stone and concrete.

It can cause dermatitis only at the manufacturing stage. The dermatitis is rare and mainly of irritant type. Only exceptionally do cobalt compounds and peroxides used in the hardening process sensitize. p-tert. Butylcatechol, which is sensitizing can be used as an inhibitor in styrene. Acrylic acid and methacrylic acid are sometimes added as solvents.

Other plastics
Polyvinyl chloride (PVC), polyethene and polystyrene hardly ever cause dermatitis. PVC contains up to 50% additives. PVC and polyethene are used in protective gloves which rarely sensitize.
Alkyd plastic (saturated polyester) is common in paint but does not sensitize.

Synthetic fibers. Nylon, perlon, terylene, dacron, acrylon, etc., are rarely allergenic. But some organic dyes are poorly fixed to these materials so that stockings, for example, can cause dermatitis.

Additives
Rare sensitizers are phthalates (dibutyl-, dioctyl- etc.), plasticizers, cobalt naphthenate, benzoyl peroxide, organic pigments, dimethyl-aniline, tricresylphoshate, resorcinol monobenzoate (UV-absorber). Resorcinol monobenzoate cross-reacts to balsam of Peru.

4.16 Preservatives, antimicrobial agents, antioxidants

Many products are chemically changed at room temperature storage by bacteria, fungi, virus, algae and oxidation. This is particularly the case when the products are water based. For this reason preservatives are added to medicaments, cosmetics, toiletries, cleansers, paints, glues, polishes, adhesives, oils, waxes, pulp, paper, cellulose and derivatives, emulsifiers, rubber, milk proofs, animal feed, food, etc.

At present it seems impossible to list completely all marketed preservatives. When information recently was collected from 21 international companies, 213 preservatives were listed. Some are marketed with different trade names and these names are sometimes changed. The preservatives are seldom labeled on the packages or mentioned in the industrial data sheets. Often the producer does not know that the raw material contains a preservative. They are in small amounts and when a product is patch tested as is or in dilution, false negative reactions often occur. Most of these biologically active substances are allergenic. Certainly allergy to these is often overlooked and may cause chronic dermatitis. Most of the preservatives have not been patch tested or examined in predictive testing.

Some of the preservatives reported to be allergenic are:
methyl-, ethyl-, propyl- and benzyl-p-hydroxybenzoates (parabens), p-chloro-m-cresol, p-chloro-m-xylenol, p-t-butylphenol, p-t-amylphenol, o-benzyl-p-chlorophenol, Irgasan DP 300, butylated hydroxyanisole (BHA), butylated hydroxytoluene (BHT), nordiguaiaretic acid (NDGA), resorcinol, pyrocatechol, phenoxyethanol, benzyl alcohol (phenylcarbinol), formaldehyde, formaldehyde releasers, quaternary ammonium salts, hydroxyquinolines, organic mercury compounds, e.g. merthiolate, phenylmercuric nitrate or acetate, hexachlorophane, 4-chlorophenol, bithionol, bromosalicylanilides, chlorosalicylanilides, trichlorocarbanilide, dichlorophene (2,2'-dihydroxy-5,5'-dichlorodiphenylmethane), chloramine, thiuramsulfides, a-naphthol, 1,3,5-tri(hydroxyethyl)-hexahydrotriazin (Grotan BK), nitrofurazone derivates, e. g. N-(5-nitrofurfuryliden-2)-3-amino-2-oxazolidone (Furazolidone), N-trichloromethylmercapto-4-cyclohexene-1, 2-dicarboximide, chloracetamide and N-methylolchloracetamide, DNCB, ethylenediamine, dithiocarbamathes. (see Formaldehyde 4,6).

Wood preservatives containing copper-chromate-arsenate compounds, pentachlorophenol, sodium pentochlorophenol, dieldrin, zinc- and copper naphthenate do not sensitize when applied in the wood. Chromate is reduced and is firmly bound. Organic tin compounds and creosote are phototoxic.
Tetrachloroisophthalonitrile is a sensitizer.

Sensitizing corrosion inhibitors in cooling water are chromate, hydrazine, ethylenediamine, mercaptobenzothiazole, triazoles. These can sometimes be replaced by nonsensitizing nitrites, silicates and phosphates.

4.17 Printing chemicals

Previously chromate, cobalt, formaldehyde, rubber chemicals, azo-dyes and photo developers were the common sensitizers in printing shops. Recently, new chemicals on the printing plates and in the inks have been marketed.

Metal or plastic sheets are coated with plastic monomers and additives. When the coating is irradiated by UV-light, the prepolymer is cured to solid material. The unirradiated parts are removed by solvents (water, ethanol, sodium hydroxide) or blown away.

The allergens are partly known; acrylate in Dycril®, penta erythrotil-tetrakis-3-mercaptopropionate and 3-mercaptopropionic acid in Letterflex®, acrylamide derivatives in Nyloprint®, N,N′-methylene-bis-acrylamide and hydroxyethylmethacrylate in NAPP®. In another process di- and tetraethylene glycol dimethacrylate have been identified as sensitizers. The sensitizer in Cyrel® seems to be unknown.

The unirradiated plate and the irradiated plate before removal of uncured material and the used solvents contain the sensitizers but the plate ready for printing is nonallergenic. The new inks contain UV-hardening acrylates (see Acrylate 4.15). They are allergenic only before irradiation.

4.18 Rubber

Four synthetic types of rubber make up about 85% of the production: butyl (isobutene/isoprene) (IIR), ethenepropene (EPM, EPDM), nitril (acrylnitril/butadien) (NBR) and chloroprene (CR) rubber.

Others are natural rubber and the synthetic styren/butadiene-(SBR), butadiene-(BR), isoprene-(IR), silicone-(Q), chlorosulfonethene-(CSM), urethane-(U), polysulfide-(T), ethenevinylacetate-(EVA), epichlorhydrine-(CO), propeneoxide-(PO), chloropolyethene-(CM), acryl-(ethylacrylate) (ACM) rubber. The main components in rubber are polymers such as plastics. When emulsified in water they form latex. Traces of catalysts, emulsifiers, etc., used at the polymerization process are present in the rubber polymer.

The rubber is delivered as a mixture of rubber/carbon black/naphthenic or aromatic oil (masterbatches). This rubber is then vulcanized (cured) to cross-link the molecular chains. To the rubber are added,depending on the type: curing agent (vulcanizer), accelerator, retardant, antioxidant, wax, sun-checking agent, peptizing agent, plasticizer, softener, rosin, resin, extenders, reinforcing agent, carbon black, filler, blowing agent, pigment, bonding agent, antitack agent, mold release agent, solvent, textile material, odorant, coupling agent. Many of these chemicals are decomposed partly or totally during the vulcanizing process, but others (for example antioxidants) are intended to be present in the cured product.

The rubber chemicals are often delivered as masterbatches: the chemicals are mixed by the producer with small amounts of rubber to prevent pollution of the dusty chemicals in the work shop.

Allergic contact dermatitis caused by rubber products is common; it is not the rubber as such which is the cause but the added rubber chemicals. The dermatitis appears not only in rubber factories but also on contact with finished rubber objects.

Sensitizing rubber chemicals:
mercaptobenzothiazole (MBT)
thiuramsulfides (TMTM, TMTD, TETD, PTD)
dithiocarbamathes (Zn-diethyl-, Zn-dibutyl-etc)
phenyl-cyclohexyl-paraphenylenediamine
dicyclohexyl-paraphenylenediamine
dimethyl-butyl-phenyl-paraphenylenediamine
diphenyl-paraphenylenediamine
diaminodiphenylmethane
isopropylaminodiphenylamine (IPPD)
diphenylguanidine (DPG)
hydroquinonemonobenzylether
dihydroxydiphenyl
hexamethylenetetramine
cyclohexyl-benzothiazole sulfenamide
diphenylthiourea
ethylene thiourea
methyl-, ethyl-, butyl thiourea
Zn/Cu compounds of thioureas

(napthylamines are now forbidden in several countries due to the risk of cancer).

The chemistry of commercial products is given in van Alphen: *Rubber Chemicals* (see References).

The rubber product which most often causes dermatitis is gloves. Rubber gloves are used in industry and especially in the household. Often they are used because of a dermatitis of another type which started on the hands. After that a secondary sensitization to rubber chemicals may occur. Other common forms of contact are via boots, shoes, tubes, handles, tires, fingerstalls, undergarments, protectors on fingers, bands, packings, adhesive tape, condoms and condom urinals.

In contact allergy against a specified rubber chemical, it is not possible to warn against any special rubber object because the added substances vary from one brand to another. Rubber gloves, however, often contain MBT, TMTM, and TMTD.

Many rubber chemicals occur not only in rubber but in other products such as plastics, pesticides, oils and organic dyes. For examples MBT can occur in antifreeze mixtures, veterinarian medicaments, insecticides, fungicides, insect repellants and in cutting oils. Diaminodiphenylmethane is used in epoxy resin systems and polyurethanes, dithiocarbamates and thiuramsulfides in pesticides. Thiuramsulfides are found in special soaps, medicaments for scabies and in Antabus®.

4.19 Tars

Coal tar and wood tars contain allergens. Coal tar is used for topical treatment and in tarred roofing and insulating tape. Creosote is a product manufactured from coal tar and used for impregnating wood. Like other tars, it is phototoxic. Wood tars are used for topical treatment. Allergy to these is often accompanied by allergy to colophony and balsams (perfume).

4.20 Turpentine

Scandinavian and Chinese turpentines are especially allergenic.

They contain hydroperoxide of 3-delta-carene. American and French turpentines contain small quantities of delta-carene. But alpha-pinene and limonene (dipentene) are allergenic and are found in all types of turpentine.

It may occur in solvents, thinners, polishes, varnishes, paints, cleansers and waxes. Previously turpentine allergy was common among painters but nowadays white spirit (kerosene) and thinner are almost exclusively used as solvents. Thinner may contain dipentene.

The term mineral turpentine is used to designate white spirit. Venice turpentine (larch turpentine) is the oleoresin from larch. It can sensitize but has no connection with the above-mentioned turpentine allergy.

Turpentine allergy is now so rare that it is no longer present in the ICDRG or NACDG routine patch test series.

4.21 Other sensitizers

Alcohols: methanol, ethanol and butanol are used as solvents in industry and laboratory work. Isopropanol occurs in cosmetics and medicaments

Aminoethylethanolamine: aluminium flux

Chloracetamide: preservative in applied medicaments, cosmetics, glues, paints

Chloramine: disinfectant

Chloroacetophenone: tear gas (Mace)

Dicyclohexyl-carbodiimide: synthesis of pharmaceutical and chemical substances

Dinitolmide: preservative in feed

Dinitrochlorobenzene (DNCB): experimental sensitizer, in coolants

Dioxane: solvent

Dodecylic aminoethyl glycine-HCl (TEGO): Disinfectant

Epichlorhydrin: in trichlorethylene used for rinsing aluminum, e. g. aircraft. The traces of epichlorhydrin present in epoxy resin rarely sensitize.

Ethoxyquin: preservative in animal foodstuffs

Ethylene glycol: solvent, antifreeze agent

Ethylene oxide: sterilizing agent

Explosives: tetryl, trinitrotoluene (TNT), dinitrotoluene (DNT), ammonium picrate, picric acid, trinitrophenol, hexanitrodiphenylamine, mercury fulminate, hydrazines

Glutaraldehyde: sterilizing agent, antiperspirant, tanning agent, fixative in electron microscopy, preservative in cosmetics and household products

Hydrazine: in cooling water, flux

Laurel oil: in perfume, spice

8-Methoxypsoralen: topical PUVA-treatment.

Octylgallate: preservative in margarine and cosmetics

Piperazine and derivatives: rubber, anthelmintic agent, epoxy hardener

Propyleneoxide: in trichlorethylene used for rinsing aluminum, e. g. in aircraft and in electron microscope work

Resorcinol monobenzoate: UV-light screening agent in plastics, e. g. glass frames

Sulfur: pesticide, medicament

Sultones and chlorosultones: contaminants in alkylethersulfates

Tetra-bishydroxy-methyl phosphonium chloride (THPC): flameproofing agent for fabrics

Tylosin tartrate: antibiotic for animals

5. Reactions to ingested allergens

There are several bases for ingested contact allergens and possibly also metal implants being able to exacerbate a current allergic contact dermatitis, but not to induce sensitization. Hand dermatitis especially seems to exacerbate from such administration. This often occurs quickly after ingestion (within a few hours) and is often of dyshidrotic palmar and plantar type.

Substances which should be particularly noted: Nickel (see Nickel 4.8.2), chromium, cobalt, photosensitizers, halogenated hydroxyquinolines, cinnamon, balsams, azodyes (e. g. tartrazine), neomycin, bacitracin, penicillin, sulfonamides, thiuram sulfides, quinine, antihistamines, p-hydroxybenzoates, propylene glycol, turpentine.

Dermatitis can be exacerbated by ingested drugs which are chemically related to skin contactants, e. g. aminophylline-/ethylenediamine, isoniazide/hydrazine, hexamethylenetetramine-/formaldehyde, antabuse/thiuram sulfides.

6. Contact urticaria syndrome

Contact urticaria is a special form of contact dermatitis. It refers to an urticarial response on exposure to certain agents. Clinically it may occur as a chronic hand dermatitis, even of vesicular type. Many, but not all, of the patients are atopics. This form of dermatitis is common in chefs, sandwich-makers and veterinarians. The mechanism may be allergic, nonallergic or uncertain. Some agents produce allergy of both immediate and delayed types, e. g. neomycin, bacitracin, penicillin, lettuce, fish and exotic woods.

6.1 Allergic contact urticaria (immediate type of hypersensitivity)

There is often a response only at the contact site; generalized urticaria, asthma and anaphylactic shock may occur after skin exposure.

Among reported agents are meat, fish, egg, flour, animal hair and dander, cow placenta, animal liver, serum and saliva, lobster, human semen, cockroaches, exotic woods, lettuce, potatoes, phenyl mercuric proprionate, benzyl alcohol, trichloroethylene, mono-amylamine (in Tolnaftate® cream), mechlorethamine hydrochloride, diethyltoluamide (insect repellent), nitrogen mustard, streptomycin, neomycin, penicillin, parabens, platinum chloride, dinitrochlorophene, Rhus, henna in hair dye.

6.2 Nonallergic contact urticaria

This is the most frequent type and can be produced in most persons.

Anaphylactic shock does not occur. The agents presumably induce release of vasoactive substances such as histamine.

Among reported agents are tetrahydrofurfuryl ester of nicotinic acid (Trafuril), cobalt chloride, cinnamic aldehyde, benzoic acid, sodium benzoate, nettles, caterpillars and dimethylsulfoxide (DMSO), ammonia.

6.3 Contact urticaria of unknown mechanism

Among reported agents are nickel- and cobalt salts, ammonium persulfate (hair bleaching agent), sorbic acid (preservative), exotic woods, polyethylene glycol, balsam of Peru, spices, cheese (contains histamine), acrylic monomer, aminophenazone, erythromycin base, denatonium benzoate (Bitrex) a denaturant in ethanol, potassium ferricyanide (photographic chemical), alcohol, formaldehyde, natural rubber latex.

6.4 Testing

Tests are performed according to a history of immediate itching, burning or stinging after contact. If there is a history of severe symptoms, one should be careful not to produce anaphylactic shock. Celery has the tendency to produce such reaction. It should be performed in a hospital with equipment for immediate treatment. Tests should be performed in controls since many substances give reactions in normal persons. The testing should be performed in this manner:

Open test is performed on the ventral forearm for 20 min and read also after 30 min and 2 hours. A positive response consists of erythema, then a wheal or wheal flare.

Occlusive patch test on the normal forearm for 20 min, should also be read after 30 min and 2 hours. A positive response is as for open test.

Occlusive patch test on recently affected skin, e. g. on the hand. A positive response consists of erythema and often vesicles.

Prick test. Only when the previous tests have failed, should prick test be performed.

One drop of the solution or the pressed juice of the product is applied to the skin. A sterile lancet is placed at an acute angle to the skin and a shallow lift made. The lancet is raised for a second before the skin is released. Any excess solution remaining on the skin after the prick has been made is removed by placing a tissue over the arm. The test sites should be 4 cm apart.

Radio allergo sorbent test (RAST) for detection of Ig E antibodies against particular allergens and the quantification of Ig E reagine antibodies may be performed.

6.5 Reactions to animal toxins

This is a special form caused by several animal organisms giving off toxins into the skin. A variety of symptoms occurs: Itch, severe burning pain, erythema, papules, vesicles, necrosis, urticaria and systemic shock. One of these conditions is Dogger Bank Itch induced by sea moss. Some algae can cause similar symptoms. Some caterpillars and moths have venomous hairs, which can pierce skin and produce nonallergic reactions. The symptoms are stinging, vesicles and sometimes local urticaria.

7. Irritant contact dermatitis

The development of irritant contact dermatitis is due both to exogenous and unexplained endogenous factors, but little is known about the pathophysiology. Probably irritants of varying chemical nature affect the skin in different ways.

From a practical point of view, two main types can be recognized; the acute and the chronic.

7.1 Irritant contact dermatitis of acute type

These reactions may vary from necrosis (corrosion) to no more than a little dryness and redness. The strength of the reaction depends on the individual susceptibility and on the concentration and chemical properties of the contactant, the presence of occlusion and the duration and frequency of exposure. Chemicals vary in their capacity to cause irritant reactions. Some will cause damage even in low concentrations while others may require high concentrations or even occlusion to elicit a response. Strong irritants cause dermatitis in nearly all individuals if there is sufficient exposure, but even with kerosene some people will fail to react to 100% strength while others will react strongly to 20%. Pigmented skin is more resistant to irritants and fair skin most susceptible. Aged skin seems to heal less readily when irritated. Some people need repeated exposure to the same skin site to give acute irritant dermatitis but others react after one exposure to the same chemical in the same concentration.

One short exposure to a chemical is sometimes sufficient to elicit an irritant reaction. This is often caused by alkalis or acids or by detergents in gloves. Alkaline dust and vapors give rise to irritant reactions on the face. When weak, the reaction disappears spontaneously in a few days. The prototype of this reaction is an irritant patch test reaction which clears spontaneously after removal of the patch test. A chemical burn is an irritant reaction which occurs mainly when working with irritant chemicals in high enough concentrations and these usually induce damage by accidental contact (see Chemical burns, 7.3).

Repeated exposure to irritants during the day, e.g. repeated handwashing, drying, cold air, may be necessary for the elicitation of the reaction, particularly leading to chapping in the winter months. Mild soaps that are tolerated in other seasons may then cause irritation. This chapping reaction, i. e. dryness and redness of the skin, disappears within a few days after treatment with a moisturizing cream.

Repeated daily exposure for weeks is usually necessary for elicitation of irritant reactions. Chapping may precede the more pronounced redness and fissuring that is characteristic of this condition. Itching is often minimal but smarting is reported. The condition is located mainly on the dorsa of the hands and the volar sides of the forearms. This type of irritant reactions occurs, for example, as the result of frequent handwashing and exposure to soluble cutting oils and shampoos or permanent wave solutions in hairdressing. In spite of the cumulative effect necessary for the development of this reaction, it may clear spontaneously when the offending causes are removed. In atopics, this type of hand dermatitis is often located on the knuckles.

In industry, irritant reactions, after single or repeated exposures, are common but are often overlooked by physicians as they clear rapidly and in most cases do not require treatment. This type of reactions is rarely described in the literature. When several factory workers develop reactions of the skin within a short period, irritant reactions should be suspected. This is in contrast to allergic contact dermatitis when one or two out of many workers exposed to relatively strong sensitizers such as epoxy resins are involved.

Some examples of acute irritant contact dermatitis:

1. A preoperative washing liquid was replaced in the winter months by a new one and 15 surgery personnel developed erythema on the dorsa of the hands and the volar sides of the forearms within a few weeks. During nonworking days the symptoms disappeared without treatment. All healed rapidly when the new washing liquid was replaced.

2. Three of four mechanics developed similar symptoms after having used a hand cleanser containing borax for a week. Again the symptoms disappeared during the weekends, and when the cleanser was replaced, no more skin reactions occurred.

3. Workers handling timber dipped in kerosene (18 % aromatics and containing preservative) developed erythema of the face and on the dorsa of their hands. There was a stinging sensation in the skin and the throat which remained throughout the night but disappeared during the weekends. When they subsequently sawed prepared but dried timber, no symptoms were elicited. The reaction was due to the timber being sawed before it was dry when the kerosene and preservative provided the volatile irritant, which was the cause of their trouble.

4. Twenty-eight out of 29 women developed chapping and redness on the dorsum of the hands within 2 weeks during the winter after having dried the hands in a warm air stream after each washing.

5. A residual solvent was demonstrated by the smell in the clothing of eight out of 10 mechanics who developed redness and dryness on the collar and wrists after having used dry-cleaned overalls. When the clothing was given a sufficient airing, the symptoms disappeared.

7.1.1 Fiberglass dermatitis

This is a type of acute irritant contact dermatitis that differs from other common irritant reactions as it is mostly papulous and itchy. The rash appears promptly after exposure. The condition occurs particularly in the building industry where glassfiber is used for insulating, textile industries where it is woven and as a reinforcement with plastics. Fibers with a diameter of less than 4.5 μ are commonly not irritating. This dermatitis is located usually on the volar side of the forearms, the collar and the waist area. When the exposure continues, the skin seems, to some extent, to become "hardened". Experience indicates that atopics have more severe symptoms than others and fail to "harden" in this way. When glass fiber fabrics are laundered in washing machines, they can contaminate other clothes and cause extensive and protracted itching among many members of the family. The fibers can be visualized with the microscope by using transparent adhesive tape to collect glass particles from the skin.

7.1.2 Newborn infant dermatitis

Newborn infants placed face downwards may (on the first to third day after delivery) develop skin irritation on protruding parts of the naked skin. The skin of the cheekbones, nose tip, chin, knees or dorsal side of the toes becomes red and often peels. The condition clears within 2–3 weeks. The irritation is caused by detergents in the textiles and by the roughness of the textile of the sheets.

7.1.3 Napkin dermatitis (diaper dermatitis)

This condition is most probably an acute irritant contact dermatitis, but is sometimes of chronic type. There is often a bacterial and yeast infection.

7.1.4 Stoma dermatitis

Irritant contact dermatitis at stoma sites are caused by the excreted material and friction from the collecting systems. These reactions tend to be rather chronic owing to continuous exposure.

7.1.5 Status eczemateous

Status eczematous, "the angry back" syndrome, "conditioned irritability", leads to a temporarily increased skin susceptibility to irritants. The skin is hyperactive and false positive patch test reactions are liable to occur. The phenomenon occurs in individuals with active dermatitis (allergic or irritant) and with strong or multiple positive patch test reactions. Otherwise tolerated chemicals which are marginal irritants (for example soap) can cause irritant reactions and patch testing with routine substances in standard concentrations can give nonspecific reactions. The status disappears when the dermatitis or test reactions are healed.

7.1.6 Stinging (subjective irritation)

Stinging may sometimes be misinterpreted as an acute irritant reaction. It is provoked by certain chemicals and is an adverse effect of many cosmetics, toiletries and topical medicaments. It occurs mainly on the face. The stinging or burning sensation or smarting arises immediately after application on the skin or with some minutes' delay. The sensation disappears within 5–15 min. There is no visible skin change. It is probably a variant of pain due to substances penetrating the skin and affecting the nerve endings. Acids, e. g. phosphoric, lactic, salicylic, sorbic, ascorbic, hydrochloric acids; alkalis, e. g. sodium hydroxide, sodium carbonate, trisodiumphosphate and other substances, e. g. aluminum compounds and propyleneglycol are the most common substances causing stinging. The irritant effect of chemicals is not synonymous with their stinging effect. Some people develop stinging more easily than others but it can be provoked in all individuals if the concentration of the chemical is increased. Sweating enhances the stinging effect. In industry and in hospitals some of the employees complain of soaps and hand lotions which are of ordinary quality. Probably many of these are "stingers". They can use other brands without trouble. The management should be aware of this phenomenon and not neglect the complaints.

7.2 Irritant contact dermatitis of chronic type (wear and tear dermatitis, traumiterative dermatitis, cumulative irritant contact dermatitis)

Irritant contact dermatitis of chronic type is as common as allergic contact dermatitis. Except in cases when the allergic symptoms are particularly pronounced, it is not possible to assess if a hand dermatitis is of allergic or irritant type by clinical examination. The connection between environment and the condition is often not so obvious as in allergic contact dermatitis. The diagnosis of irritant contact dermatitis is commonly established when there is no explainable positive patch test reaction and there are possible contacts with irritants.

The endogenous predisposition is decisive and probably even more pronounced than in allergic contact dermatitis or in the irritant contact dermatitis of acute type. Contact allergy can be experimentally induced in most individuals by at least strong sensitizers at sufficient exposure and irritant reactions of acute type can be elicited in nearly all individuals if the exposure to an irritant is sufficient. The irritant contact dermatitis of chronic type, however, is able to be elicited only in some individuals. Thus, only a few workers who are heavily exposed for years to irritants develop irritant dermatitis of chronic type. In contrast to this, many of those who develop irritant contact dermatitis on the hands have been exposed to rather weak irritants, e. g. in common wet work, for as little as a couple of weeks or months. Also chemicals which in 100% concentrations fail to produce irritant reactions under occlusion, e. g. acetone and ethanol, may do so after repeated exposure.

Contact irritant dermatitis sometimes starts under rings or on the thin skin of the interdigital clefts with dryness, fissures and redness, often followed by swelling and vesicle formation.

The dermatitis is located mainly on the dorsa of the hands and fingers and sometimes on the forearms. Later the condition may spread to the volar aspect of the hand. Isolated localization to the volar sides is rare. Cases with only one hand affected are also rare in contrast to cases of the acute type. When exposure to the suspected irritant has been eliminated, the dermatitis in many cases does not clear spontaneously. Once the dermatitis has become established, even cold, heat, mechanical insults, secondary infections and mild irritants can perpetuate the condition or cause relapses in skin which, to the naked eye, seems to be healed. This may continue for months or years, even with topical corticosteroid treatment.

The pathological process is of an unknown nature but seems to be able to "repeat itself" once started. How this process is different from that occuring in the acute type is unknown. Hypothetically there is a defect repair mechanism.

Clinical observations indicate that those with an "atopic constitution" are more prone to develop irritant contact dermatitis. In several reports, 15–20 % of patients with this type of irritant contact dermatitis have a history of atopy. However, the atopic constitution in a population is considered to be in the same range so the evidence of correlation is not free from objection. The endogenous factor is obvious but cannot be predicted.

The irritant contact dermatitis of chronic type occurs in nearly all kinds of occupations except office work, where the working environment is mostly dry and clear.

7.3 Chemical burns

Some chemicals have the capacity to cause such strong irritant reactions that a chemical burn (corrosion) appears. It involves a direct chemical action on normal living cells that results in disintegration at the site of contact corresponding to what occurs with thermal burns. The effect on the skin is due to the nature of the chemical, the concentration and the exposure time. Occlusion enhances the effect. Chemicals which do not give even a slight irritant effect when applied open, can corrode under occlusion, as happens when kerosene, acids or alkalis enter gloves through a hole or above the cuff.

By and large, the development of a chemical burn is a sequel to accidental exposure. Therefore the connection between the injurious substance and the injury is easily proven.

The skin condition is sharply limited to the contact area, has no tendency to spread and stings or smarts more than itches. Often the burn appears within seconds or minutes, but sometimes the development is delayed for several hours. For example, a chemical burn on the knees after contact with fresh concrete appears within 8–12 hours and may become worse over the following 24 hours. This is also the case when, for example, alkalis or acids have entered gloves.

Usually the burn looks red and swollen. Acids mostly give a crust but alkalis often form blisters or vesicles and pustules. The chemical burn from fresh concrete often gives a dark brown crust. Phenol (carbolic acid) makes the skin white, wrinkled and softened and later causes a crust. There is no pain immediately but intense burning is felt later, followed by local anesthesia. Sometimes a deep necrosis develops. Cresol and chlorinated phenols, common in industry, give the same severe chemical burns.

Hydrofluoric acid gives painful reactions as fluorine binds calcium in the tissues. When it is used in lower concentrations, there is no immediate reaction but absorption continues, for example from the cuticles, and painful deep reactions may appear several hours later.

Many other chemically active substances can cause chemical burns. The most severe manifestations are ulceration and scars.

8. Common irritants

8.1 Water

If the surface film and horny layer have been damaged by solvents, detergents, etc., water can dissolve the water-binding substances in the horny layer and cause dryness. Water is hypotonic and can be toxic to the living epidermal cells. Calcium, magnesium and iron in hard water can be deposited in the skin cracks and cause mechanical and chemical irritation. High concentrations of chlorine in swimming pools can irritate. If the water is permitted to act for a long time a maceration takes place and the possibilities for harmful substances to penetrate are increased.

8.2 Skin cleansers

Soap does not seem harmful to normal skin, but if the skin has previously been damaged, the soap can have an irritant effect. Abrasives in soaps often have more damaging effect than the soap itself. Certain so-called water-free cleansers containing solvents have a more powerful effect on the skin. In many occupations where the skin gets dirty, the cleansers – especially in the form of organic solvents or alkalis – cause considerably greater damage to the skin than the work itself.

8.3 Cleansers

Detergents and dish – washing liquids in concentrations prescribed by the manufacturer have a fairly mild effect on normal skin. Most often such substances are used in too high a concentration in the suds. When detergents as powder are added to washing machines and dishwashers, the hands are easily contaminated. They work first by dissolving fat and water-binding substances. When they penetrate deeper, they denature the protein and damage cell membranes. Proteolytic enzymes in detergents can irritate. Certain perfumes in detergents may act as irritants when dissolved in hot water.

8.4 Alkalis

The most common are soap, soda, ammonium, potassium and sodium hydroxide, cement, lime, sodium silicate, trisodium phosphate and different types of amine (e.g. epoxy resin hardeners), stearylamine (emulsifier), monoethanol amine in antirust agents. They dissolve the skin's fat and water binding substances and break the chemical chains in the keratin. Alkalis are used in many industries, such as dyeing, tanning, and manufacturing of plastics and glass. Certain copying processes use ammonium, which is vaporized and can cause irritation on the face. Soda ash (anhydrous sodium carbonate) is three times stronger than common washing soda.

8.5 Acids

Diluted acids generally damage the skin less than the corresponding concentrations of alkalis. Strong concentrations of, e.g. hydrochloric acid, nitric acid, chromic acid, hydrofluoric acid, are used in many industries and can cause corrosion of the skin. Organic acids (e.g. oxalic acid) are present in some plants and bulbs. Among saturated free fatty acids, particularly C_8 through C_{12} are irritating.

8.6 Oils

Soluble cutting oils and coolants contain oil, water and emulsifiers and also antioxidants, anticorrosion agents, preservatives and sometimes perfume. Through their emulsifying effect they dry out the skin. Sulfated and chlorinated oils are more irritating.

Lubricating oils and hydraulic oils are generally difficult to remove. The consequence is that one is often forced to use organic solvents to get the hands clean, which can further worsen the injury.

8.7 Organic solvents

These are extensively used in many industries. The most common are white spirit, benzene, toluene, aromatic petroleum solvents, trichloroethylene (TRI), perchlorethylene (PER), methylene chloride, trichlorethane (methylchloroform) chlorobenzene, methanol, ethanol, isopropanol, propylene glycol, ethylacetate, acetone, methylethylketone, nitroethane, and carbon disulfide.

Thinner often consists of a mixture of alcohols, ketones and sometimes toluene and dipentene (sensitizer). The aromatic solvents especially irritate the skin. White spirit (kerosene) contains 18% aromatics and primegrade kerosene 2%, sometimes down to 0.1%.

In cleansing from oil, a mixture of solvents and detergents is used. Solvents which are not completely removed from for example working clothing after waterless cleansing can irritate the skin on legs, wrists and neck.

8.8 Oxidants

Hydrogen peroxide and especially organic peroxides, e.g. benzoyl peroxide and cyclohexanon peroxide, are used in several industries including the production of polyester plastic products. Organic peroxides may occur in flour and perborate in washing powders.

8.9 Reducing agents

Thioglycolates are used in permanent waving of hair. They break the chemical links between the keratin molecules, allowing the keratin to swell and thereby increase the penetration possibilities.

8.10 Plants

Orange peel and hyacinth and tulip bulbs contain irritants, as do pineapple juice, cucumbers, asparagus, mustard, barley and corn, spurge, pasque flower, wind flower, rice, bamboo.

8.11 Animal substances

Enzymes which come onto the skin when the pancreas is being removed from the intestines in slaughterhouses can damage the skin and cause onycholysis. Feces, urine and the intestinal contents from colostomies can have an irritant effect. Fish and shrimp are irritating. Butchers develop irritation on the forearms due to friction of the pigs' skin and possibly fatty acids.

8.12 Other organic substances

Formaldehyde, allyl alcohol, cyanoacrylate in glue, cresol, chloro-cresols and -phenols, occur in pesticides, alkyl bromides in pain killers, styrene in plastic monomers and halogenated acetophenones in tear gas (Mace). Alkyl-tin compounds (TBTO) are used as preservatives for wood and textiles.

Compounds with unsaturated chains are irritants, e.g. allyl alcohol and -aldehyde, diallyl-phthalate and -glycol and croton-aldehyde.

8.13 Medicaments for local treatment

Tar, potassium permanganate, gentian violet, hexachlorophene, quaternary ammonium compounds, mercury preparations, ant-hralin can – especially if they are used in high concentrations – cause "overtreatment dermatitis". Occlusive treatment magnifies this potential.

8.14 Other inorganic substances

Bromine, chlorine, mercury salts and zinc chlorides or phosphoric acid in solders, sodium bifluoride in flux and wood preservatives and antimony trioxide are irritants.

8.15 Physical and mechanical factors

Heat, steam, cold, sunshine, ultraviolet light and other radiations are irritating to the skin. Friction, pressure and scratching of the skin can cause increased permeability. Metal particles, adhesive plaster, insulating tape, glass wool, particles of textiles, sawdust, sand, asbestos, cement and plaster can cause an increase in permeability mechanically.

8.16 Cosmetics

Mascara preparations, face creams, antiperspirants (aluminum chlorhydroxide is less irritant than aluminum chloride), deodorants with quaternary ammonium compounds, propellants in hygiene sprays, cleaning solutions, may be irritants. Propylene glycol is an irritant.

8.17 Carbonless paper (NCR paper)

NCR (No Carbon Required, National Cash Register) can cause irritation on the face and the hands/arms probably owing to solvents released when the small capsules containing dye are broken at writing.

8.18 Plastic low molecular material

Several monomers and cross-linking substances are sensitizers and irritants. Particularly irritating are acrylates, phenol-formaldehyde resins, isocyanates, diallylphthalate, diallyl glycol carbonate, styrene. The epoxy oligomers of bisphenol A type are weak or non irritants.

9. Photo contact dermatitis

9.1 Photoallergic contact dermatitis (Test substances: see 22.5)

Photoallergy involves an immunological process and occurs only after an incubation period. Cross-reactions with immunochemically closely related substances are not unusual. Small amounts of daylight which normally reach the skin can be sufficient to provoke a reaction. Common fluorescent tubes give off a certain amount of UV-light.

The photoallergic contact dermatitis with erythema, infiltration, papules/vesicles occurs in skin areas that have been in contact with photosensitizing substances and that have been illuminated with sunlight within the preceding 24 h. The most common localization is the face, a triangle on the upper part of the chest and the back of the hands and forearms. On the face there is often a clear patch beneath the eyebrows, nose and chin. The skin is unaffected on a triangle behind the ears and under watchstraps and spectacles. This dermatitis can, like allergic contact dermatitis, spread secondarily to other unexposed areas. Photoallergic contact dermatitis and airborne allergic contact dermatitis, for example from Chrysanthemum plants, can imitate each other. Another differential diagnosis is actinic reticuloid.

Many photoallergic substances in a higher concentration also cause phototoxic reactions. Exceptions are 6-methylcoumarin and PABA.

A certain proportion of afflicted persons develop "persistent light sensitivity", that is, they are sensitive to UV-light for months or years without any apparent contact with the offending chemical.

Among photoallergic substances are:

Drugs such as phenothiazines (chlorpromazines, promethazin), sulfonamides, chlorosalicylamide (antifungal), dichlorophene, dihydroxy-dichloro-diphenylsulfide (antifungal), diphenhydramine, quinidine.

Antimicrobial agents such as chloro- and bromosalicylanilides, bithionol, fentichlor, hexachlorophene.

Sunscreening agents such as para-aminobenzoates, digalloyl oleate, benzophenones, cinnamates.

Quinine in hair lotions and soft drinks.

Plants, e.g. lichens.

Quindoxin (quinoxaline di-N-oxide), growth promoting factor in pig feed.

Dimethylthiourea in photocopy paper.

Perfume substances, 6-methylcoumarin, sandalwood oil, musk ambrette.

9.2 Phototoxic reactions

Certain substances cause a reaction only if the skin is exposed, after their absorption, to ultraviolet light. Similar reactions may occur when the phototoxic substance has been ingested.

Like the irritants the phototoxic substances may cause a reaction in all people after the first contact – if they are present in a strong enough concentration for a long enough time and if enough ultraviolet light energy is added. The strength of the reaction varies among different people.

The reaction is usually of the same type as that seen with strong exposure to the sun, i.e. reddening with subsequent pigmentation. Sometimes the reaction is so severe that vesicles and bullae appear.

Not infrequently large bullae occur in the form of lines on the body on people who have been in contact with the wild meadow parsnip and at the same time have been sunbathing (meadow grass dermatitis).

Among phototoxic substances should particularly be mentioned:

Drugs for systemic use. Barbiturates, tetracyclines (e.g. demethylchlortetracycline, oxycycline), phenothiazines (chlorpromazine), psoralens, nalidixic acid, griseofulvin, sulfonamides and related compounds.

Topical phototoxic substances.

Tars, pitch and *creosote* (in wood preservatives).

Furocoumarins (psoralens) are present in plants and plant products, and cause "phytophoto dermatitis", e.g. lemon peel, fennel, dill, angelica, fig, buttercup, carrots, parsnips, celery, bergamot oil and other volatile oils.

Dyes such as eosin, acridine, fluorescein and rose bengale.

Cadmium sulfide in tattoos can cause a reaction.

Tributyltinoxide (TBTO) is a preservative for wood, textiles, etc.

10. Patch testing

(Test substances: see 22.)

The purpose of patch testing is to discover a contact allergy. It is performed by placing suspected allergens on normal skin in the correct way and in a suitable concentration. If an eczematous reaction is provoked, the person has a contact allergy to the tested substance.

Patch testing is indicated in suspected allergic contact dermatitis when the cause is unknown or uncertain. The indication can be weaker if the case history and examination point to a definite allergen. If the clinical course is drawn out, patch testing is indicated even if some allergen is known to be the main cause, as it can happen that there is a simultaneous allergy to another less obvious allergen. Clinical impressions can be misleading. It is often difficult to find a connection between dermatitis and allergens which are present in everyday life, e.g. nickel, chromate, rubber, dyes, perfumes. This applies especially for hand dermatitis where there is generally an indication for patch testing. Stasis dermatitis is often complicated by contact allergy to topical drugs. Atopic dermatitis, seborrhoeic dermatitis and nummular dermatitis generally do not indicate patch testing but such patients can sometimes be sensitized secondarily to topical medicaments. Cement-chromate dermatitis may simulate nummular dermatitis on the hands.

Preemployment testing with potential sensitizers in a new job should not be performed.

Patch testing is contraindicated in acute or widespread dermatitis since the dermatitis may get worse and nonspecific test reactions can be provoked. The test site should be free from dermatitis for at least 1 month. Corrosives and chemicals with a potential systemic effect should be tested with caution.

Systemic treatment with less than 15 mg/day of prednisolone does not, as a rule, prevent test reactions appearing.

When selecting test substances one should choose the substances with which the patient is in contact. It is often impossible to find out which those are, as the most common allergens are spread throughout the everyday environment. For these reasons it has become more common in most countries to use a standard test series (battery). The selection of these routine substances must be adapted to the local occurrence of specific industrial products, medicaments and plants. Testing with a standard series is not sufficient in itself but must be supplemented with additional substances in accordance with the patient's case history. As a contaminant in a product can be the the sensitizer, it is important to use the actual batch.

The best all purpose vehicle is petrolatum. Some substances, however, dissolve in water, e.g. metal salts and formaldehyde. Turpentine is soluble in olive oil. Petrolatum is not a suitable vehicle for chromate, chlorhexidine, acrlylates and PABA. The patient's own materials can sometimes be dissolved in water, alcohol, methylethylketone (MEK) or acetone; otherwise petrolatum is used. Solid substances such as cloth, plants (some are irritants!) and rubber can be applied as they are. Sometimes positive test reaction can be achieved only from extracts of leather, textiles, rubber, etc. The substance is extracted with acetone or alcohol over a period of 15–20 min at 40°–50°C.

The concentration of the test substances is of fundamental important for the test results. Standard test substances in routine concentrations generally do not provoke irritant reactions, but they can in certain circumstances and in some persons cause false positive or false negative reactions. With regard to the patient's own materials, an open test with different concentrations should be used first. If the result is negative, a patch test can be performed with 10–100 times lower concentration. A suitable concentration for patch testing is for most substances 0.1–1.0%. Most medicaments and cosmetics may be applied as they are, but there is a risk of false negative reactions. Testing with the ingredients is therefore often necessary. Some preparations may be applied after the irritant solvent has evaporated. Children below 15 should be tested with half strength, as they are prone to give irritant reactions.

For psychological reasons it is recommended not to test pregnant women. A later abortion may be related to the test performance by the patient.

Storage of the test preparations must be done in such a way that they do not get contaminated by foreign substances or change their concentration. Dissolved substances must be kept in glass bottles with a stopper that must not be of rubber. Petrolatum preparations are best kept in disposable plastic syringes or plastic sqeeze bottles.

The test patches should be applied on the back and outer side of the upper part of the arms. A well-fitting, nonporous tape is used. If the test unit and the adhesive tape do not give full and complete occlusion, as much as 40% false negative test reactions can be obtained.

Before application, the skin must not be locally treated with soap, solvents or have tape applied. When the adhesive tape with the test units has been applied, marking must be done at the side of each test patch. That can be done with (1) fluorescein sodium or (2) dihydroxyacetone 20 g – water 50 ml – washable ink 5 ml – acetone ad 100 ml, or (3) pyrogallol 5 g – ferric (III) chloride saturated in water 8 ml – acetone 20 ml – ethanol 40 ml or gentian violet. If test strips with constant distance between filter paper discs are used, only one marking is needed, at one end of the strip.

The patient should understand the nature of the investigation, therefore some information should be given. The following instructions are recommended:

> To establish whether you are allergic to certain materials or substances, a series of patch tests have been applied to your skin. These patch tests may identify the cause of an allergic dermatitis.
> The patch tests must be left in place for 2 days and 2 nights. During this time or some days later a red area about 10–15

mm in size may appear; it may itch.

As a rule, such reactions indicate that you are allergic to the corresponding substances.

In order to increase the reliability of the tests, the following precautions should be observed:

(1) You should not bathe, shower or wash the back where the patch tests are applied.
(2) Avoid excessive exercise which causes heavy sweating.
(3) Avoid friction or rubbing of the patch tests as this may cause them to become loose.
(4) Avoid scratching the areas where redness and itching appear.
(5) Do not expose the test area to the sun or ultraviolet lamp.
(6) Should the patch test or adhesive tape become loose, apply additional tape to the patch test so that it is refixed to the original area. Please report to your doctor on the next visit that you had to refix the test patch.
(7) If you observe a reaction at the test site within 3 weeks of your visit to the doctor, you must report it as it may be important.

The reading of the result should take place no earlier than several hours but preferably 24 h after the patches have been removed.

Sometimes it is advisable for the patient to remove the adhesive tape after 2 days and for the first reading to be made on the third day after the application. In such a case the skin marking must be made at the time of application. A fresh reading should be taken after a further 2 days. Certain substances, e.g. neomycin and organic dyes, cause reactions which may not appear until after 4–6 days. To avoid false negative reactions, a last reading should be done 7 days after application.

An allergic test reaction is characterized by itching, erythema, papules, infiltration and possibly vesicles. It should always be possible to palpate the infiltration. Often there is a reaction outside the area where the test substance has been applied, and therefore the boundary is diffuse. The reaction remains for several days and can sometimes increase in strength after removal. The feature of test reactions is partly due to the test substance. Thus, nickel often gives vesicles in weak reactions but PPD and PPD derivatives (rubber chemicals) give more pronounced infiltration. The test reaction does not always have the same appearance as the clinical dermatitis because of the latter being altered by time, treatment and substances other than the provoking allergen.

Irritant test reaction exists in several types. The skin becomes red with a brown hue, sharply delimited to the application area of the test substance. It is typical that there is no itching, infiltration, papules or vesicles. Most irritant reactions appear within 1 day, but "delayed irritant" reactions to certain acrylates have been observed. An irritant reaction of this type which is not particularly strong weakens and disappears in about a day. On patch testing with alkali, soap and detergents, the skin often becomes swollen without simultaneous erythema ("glazed reaction"). Sometimes there may be an erosion or a bulla. There can be an irritant reaction which looks like a contact allergic reaction and cannot be distinguished from one by the naked eye. That is the case with quaternary ammonium compounds, for example.

Sensitizers used in concentrations near the irritating limit, e.g. turpentine, formaldehyde, tars, quaternary ammonium compounds, benzoylperoxide, phenol-formaldehyde resins, sometimes give reactions which should be suspected to be of an irritant type. Reactions to substances that even in 100% concentration do not give irritant reactions can with greater certainty be considered as allergic.

When several reactions are obtained, particularly weak ones should be suspected to be irritant on an "angry back" (see 7.1.5). They should be retested separately 1–2 weeks later.

If the reaction is suspected to be of irritant type, the testing should be repeated with the substance diluted 2–10 times. When patch tests are performed with unknown substances, it is best to do an open test first. Substances that have not been described as allergens and that have caused a reaction with signs of allergic reaction should be tested on at least 20 healthy persons, so that one can decide if it is an allergic reaction. Owing to the great individual variation of susceptibility to irritants, 20 are not always sufficient. It would generally be difficult for nondermatologists to make such an examination.

Pustular patch test reactions are clinically distinct from allergic and irritant reactions. The pustules are 1–3 mm in diameter. They are produced by heavy metals, nickel, mercury, arsenic, in both atopic and other individuals but are rare. Often they cannot be reproduced by repeated testing. Recording of test reactions is proposed as follows:

+? doubtful reaction; faint erythema only

+ weak positive reaction; erythema, infiltration, possibly papules

++ strong positive reaction; erythema, infiltration, papules, vesicles

+++ extreme positive reaction; intense erythema and infiltration and coalescing vesicles

− negative reaction

IR Irritant reaction of different types

NT not tested

The time after application should be given in days, e.g. D2, D3, D5 (D = days after application). Reactions developing on D7 or later are regarded as late reactions, i.e. test sensitization.

A false positive reaction implies that the test response seems positive in the absence of contact allergy. This means that these reactions are of irritant type.

A false negative reaction means that patch testing has failed to provoke a positive reaction despite the presence of contact allergy. The cause of missing reactions can of course be that the patient has not been tested with the correct allergen. A false negative reaction in the true sense of the term is said to be present if an allergic patient does not react positively to the patch test performed with the allergen.

10.1 False negative reactions
The level of sensitivity is low

The test concentration is too low
The amount of test substance is too small
The test substance is of the wrong composition
The vehicle does not release the test substance
The occlusion is insufficient
The test site is on the wrong area
The reading is made too early
Local corticosteroid depresses or delays the reaction
Systemic corticosteroid depresses or delays the reaction
Testing in a refractory phase
The test has not been in place long enough, has fallen off or slipped.
The test does not reproduce the clinical exposure with adjuvant factors present.
Cytostatic agent might depress the reaction
No UV irradiation in photo sensitivity

A formulated product may give positive reaction but all the ingredients give negative reactions. There are several reasons for this: The reaction was of irritant type. A contaminant in the actual batch of the product is the sensitizer but is not present in the testing ingredients. The penetration of the sensitizer into the skin is enhanced by other ingredients. The sensitizer is not released from the vehicle used.

10.2 False positive reactions

Too high concentration for the patient being tested
The test substance is contaminated by an irritant
The vehicle is irritant
Too much test substance has been applied
The test in unevenly dispersed with spots with too high concentration
The test substance has become concentrated to the edges of the patch for physical reasons
Application on the wrong test area
An acute dermatitis is present
Dermatitis present near the test site
The patient has an irritable skin without visible dermatitis

The test site was recently affected by dermatitis
The test site has recently been used for patch testing
Pressure effect of solid material
Strong adhesive tape reaction
The test material has caused the reaction
The test is unevenly dispersed with spots of too high concentration

10.3 Explanation of patch test reactions

A true positive allergic test reaction indicates that the person tested has been exposed and sensitized to the test allergen. The test substance may be a single chemical, or the response may be to one chemical in a test mixture, or it may be a cross-reaction; 10–20% of adults without dermatoses give positive test reactions.

The reaction may be expected and is then easy to explain.

Some unexpected reactions to substances in the standard series may be explained by renewed inquiry into the patient's history or possibly by examination of the patient's environment, e.g. place of work.

The following points should be considered when explaining the significance of the reactions:

Reaction explained by the actual dermatitis. Judging from the patient's history and the localization, contact with the substance in question has occurred in relation to the present episode of dermatitis.

Reaction explained by previous episode of dermatitis. The test substance in question has caused previous dermatitis but does not explain the present episode.

Reaction without explanation. The reasons may be the following:
1. Lack of knowledge on the part of the examiner.
2. Some sources of the substance in question have not been traced.
3. The patient has not given sufficient information on contactants, partly perhaps because of the inability of the examiner to ask the proper questions. The patient may have forgotten a previous history of dermatitis to personal nickel objects, for example.
4. The substance occurs widely in the environment so that a significant contact cannot be clarified by history. Such

substances are nickel, chromium, cobalt, formaldehyde, colophony, balsams, tars.

5. The patient has never developed dermatitis from the substance as he has not been exposed to sufficient amounts after sensitization.
6. Contact has occurred with a cross-reacting substance, which may have a different usage.

10.4 Risks of testing

Patch testing involves a certain risk of sensitization or raising of the level of sensitivity. The sensitization manifests itself as a "late reaction" (flare-up) in a small number of cases. Certain substances sometimes induce patch test sensitization, e.g. poison ivy, *Primula obconica,* streptomycin, reactive diluents for epoxy resins, beryllium and azo-compounds (dyes and rubber chemicals). Photo patch tests also involve risk of sensitization, e.g. chlorpromazines. If testing with these substances is considered necessary, they should be applied in low concentrations.

Other disadvantages of patch testing include the reactions themselves if they are strong and in some cases secondary local depigmentation from certain phenols (preservatives in oils and soaps, etc., and phenol-formaldehyde resins) and pigmentation from certain perfumes and optical whiteners.

Anaphylactic shock has been described to neomycin and bacitracin, for example (see Contact urticaria, 6.)

10.5 Open test

In the open test, absorption is not increased by occlusion. In cases with a high degree of allergy a sufficient amount can be absorbed. It is recommended as a first test on unknown substances and products which the patient brings. The test substance should be dissolved in a volatile solvent such as ether, acetone, alcohol, butylacetate. Also solvents which produce an irritant reaction in the closed patch test may be used safely. Cosmetics or topical medicaments may be applied as they are. The test solution is dropped onto the skin and allowed to spread by itself. The time for reading and the characteristics of the reaction are the same as with closed patch testing.

10.6 Usage test (Provocative test)

This repeated open test is used preferably for topical medicaments and cosmetics. The preparation is applied in a thin layer on the volar forearm twice dayly for 5 days. The preparations may be applied for 3 to 5 days at the site of a previous dermatitis. A reaction is not necessarily of allergic type but may be an irritant.

10.7 Testing of oral mucosa

Such testing is unreliable.

10.8 Intradermal testing

This technique has been recommended for some allergens which are not always absorbed in sufficient quantities on patch testing, e.g. neomycin, gentian violet, merthiolate, rivanol, penicillin and metal salts (Cr, Ni, Co). The metal salts are used in a concentration of 0.01 and $0.001 \ mol \cdot lit^{-1}$. The test reaction is most intense on D2. If the patch test is performed with good occlusion, there is rarely any need to use intradermal testing.

Flow chart for patch testing

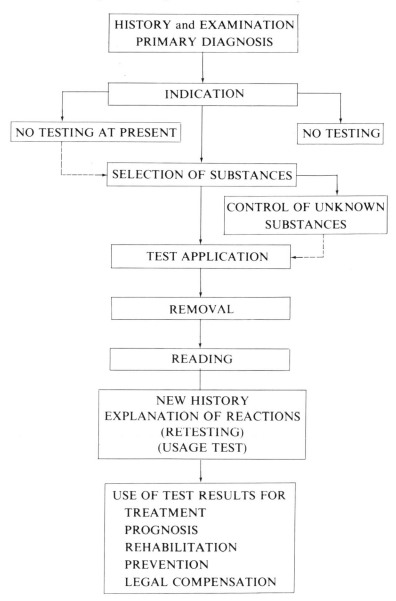

11. Photo patch testing

(Test substances: see 22.5)

A Xenon lamp is the best light source but for practical use fluorescent tubes are recommended. Using window glass as a filter, only long wave (> 320 nm) light is obtained. This light source can also be used for photo testing.

The source consists of four fluorescent lamps (24″ tubes): two with short wave UV light and two with long wave:

"Sunlamps" (280–355 nm; max. 310 nm)

Westinghouse Sunlamps FS 20 T 12

"Blacklights" (320–440 nm; max. 350 nm)

Westinghouse F 20 T 12 BLB

General Electric F 20 T 12 BLB

The two different types of tubes are mounted alternately, 10 mm from each other, in a box with a 15×30 cm opening that can be protected with a 2 mm thick window glass. This opening should be 15 cm from the tubes. Behind them there should be a light-reflecting aluminum plate.

For irradiation of the photo patch test only UV light is used, which has a wavelength of more than 320 nm, obtained by filtration with window glass. This light produces no reaction on normal skin, so that it is not necessary to screen off the light from the areas not tested.

Sufficient irradiation of the photo patch test with filtered light takes about 15 minutes. The actual optimal period must be calculated separately for each type of equipment.

Before photo patch testing-or at the same time – the following should be established by photo testing: the MED (minimal erythema dose) read after 1 day (< 320 nm) is normal, the MED causes only erythema, long wave UV light (> 320 nm) does not elicit skin reaction.

Two identical closed patch tests using the same test substance are applied simultaneously; both are adequately covered with black paper or a nontransparent test patch. One of the patches is removed after 1 day. Before irradiation all excess substance and petrolatum should be removed by washing with a suitable solvent so that the test substance does not act like a sunscreen on the skin surface.

Preparations which the patient brings can best be applied first as an open test; he can then expose himself to sunlight.

The test site is irradiated with long wave UV light. The results are read after a further day. At the same time the second test (plain patch test) is removed and if the reaction is negative, the area is immediately covered with nontransparent material, e.g. black paper, to protect it from light. The results are read after a further 1–2 days.

Positive photo patch test reactions resemble plain patch test responses. Photoallergic and contact allergic reactions may occur simultaneously to the same test substance.

If photoallergy to a drug given systemically is suspected, the therapeutic dose may be given for 2 days before irradiation. A 1–2 cm² area bordered by black nontransparent paper should be irradiated. The results are read after a further 2 days.

The photo patch test reactions are recorded in the same way as plain test reactions:

Ph?+	doubtful reaction; faint erythema only
Ph+	weak positive reaction; erythema, infiltration, possibly papules
Ph++	strong positive reaction; erythema, infiltration, papules, vesicles
Ph+++	extreme positive reaction; intense erythema and infiltration and coalescing vesicles
Ph−	negative reaction
Ph T	phototoxic reaction
Ph NT	not photo patch tested

Indications for photo patch testing should preferably be limited to those patients whose dermatitis raises suspicion of photo allergic contact dermatitis.

12. Points in differential diagnosis

(See also allergic contact dermatitis 3.2, irritant contact dermatitis 7., photoallergic contact dermatitis 9.1).

Especially after a lapse of time it is impossible to differentiate between allergic and irritant contact dermatitis on the hands. Both types are often present at the same time on this location. Furthermore several chemicals are both irritants and sensitizers.

Photoallergic dermatitis and phototoxic dermatitis on the face normally differ from airborne allergic contact dermatitis in that the regions round the eyes and under the nose and chin in the former cases are left free. Allergic contact dermatitis on the face often affects the area around the eyes with swelling of the eyelids.

Sometimes a thermal or chemical burn or wound does not heal but a dermatitis develops around the damaged site. Then there is a spreading of the dermatitis often of nummular type on the body.

Plant dermatitis on the face can resemble atopic dermatitis and photoallergic dermatitis.

Seborrhoeic dermatitis on the face and axillae may be difficult to distinguish from contact dermatitis. On the face it normally occurs round alae nasi, in the eyebrows and behind the ears.

Paronychia may be of primary origin or secondary to dermatitis.

"Dyshidrotic eczema" (pompholyx, vesiculosis,) with repeated eruptions of itching vesicles on finger sides and volae may resemble allergic contact dermatitis particularly from nickel.

Psoriasis on the palms without engagement of the body otherwise may be impossible to distinguish from allergic contact dermatitis caused by, e.g. tires or rubber handles.

Trichophyton rubrum on the palms of the hands may be difficult to distinguish from contact dermatitis and psoriasis.

Cement dermatitis may look like nummular dermatitis on the back of the hands.

Pustulosis on the palms may resemble infected hand dermatitis.

Lesions such as lichen planus may appear in allergic contact dermatitis caused by p-phenylenediamine derivatives in color developers.

Phenylisopropyl-p-phenylenediamine in rubber may cause purpura.

Early porphyria cutanea tarda may simulate a bullous allergic contact dermatitis on the back of the hands.

Atopic dermatitis and allergic contact dermatitis caused by nickel in the fold of the elbow may look alike.

Leg eczema is often primarily or secondarily caused by contact allergy to local medication.

"Athlete's foot" and foot dermatitis from shoes and socks may resemble each other.

Erysipelas, dermatomyositis, polymorphic light eruption and Quincke's edema should be differentiated from allergic contact dermatitis on face and hands.

Vesicles on the palms from caterpillars may simulate vesiculous allergic contact dermatitis.

Generalized erythroderma secondary to allergic contact dermatitis may be impossible to differentiate from other forms of this condition.

Papular drug eruption on the body may simulate textile dermatitis.

Scabies in an extensive stage may resemble papulo/vesiculous contact dermatitis.

13. Occupational contact dermatitis

Occupational contact dermatitis can be defined medically as contact dermatitis for which exposure at work can be shown to be the main cause or one of the factors contributing to its occurrence.

From the legal point of view some forms are excluded, but the rules vary from country to country.

Conditions to which attention should be paid in an investigation of suspected occupational dermatitis are:
1. There has been contact with substances known to cause dermatitis. Both products that have been present for years and those that have been introduced recently may be the cause.
2. Presence of similar types of dermatitis in others employed at the same plant. But even in fairly large work groups only occasional sensitization to a particular substance except, for example, exotic woods and epoxy resin is usually seen. Where there are many affected at the same time at a work site, it is more probable that the condition is irritant reaction rather than allergic.
3. The existence of a time link between exposure and occurrence. Sometimes allergic dermatitis is provoked no sooner than 4–5 days after contact. Renewed exposure once a week may cause a stationary dermatitis. The time link can be difficult to establish.
4. Appearance and localization coincide with other definite cases. However, if there are several factors contributing to the occurrence, the appearance may alter. Localization is usually on the hands without any specific appearance.
5. Attacks occur when at certain jobs, while improvement can be

seen when at other jobs or when on sick leave, holidays or weekends. Often the maintaining factors are present even in the off-work environment, which is the case with chromium, nickel and rubber.

6. When there is a link between the history and positive test reactions, this is strong proof.

7. It happens sometimes that 10–20% of the employees complain of occupational skin diseases. It is then wise to perform a site visit and examine all complainants. The result is often that one or two have an occupational skin disease and the others common skin diseases. The basis for the complaint is often "psychologic disturbance" at the site.

8. One may believe that automatic processes imply safety as regards contact between chemicals and skin, but there are many possibilities for contact, e.g. delivery of raw material, storage in contaminated drums and sacks, weighing of chemicals, charging of dyes, preservatives, etc., sampling of process material for control, laboratory controls, leakage on floor, vessels, taps, etc., cleaning of vessels, repair, mending of final product, waste materials.

Several circumstances may cause legal problems:

1. It is sometimes clear in a particular case that factors deriving from the physical constitution are of great importance. Persons with, for example, atopic dermatitis in childhood, seem to develop an irritant hand dermatitis in wet or dirty work. The importance of the occupational factors, however, is obvious when it is known that these people usually do not get dermatitis when working in an office.

2. Previously existing conditions may become worse through work. Thus a ring dermatitis which has been fairly slight for many years with complete healing periodically may become worse after continuous cleaning work.

3. Severe exacerbation of a slight nonincapacitating, irritant dermatitis occurs through secondary sensitization to topical medication which the doctor has prescribed or the patient has used on his own.

4. A person in his free time may have become sensitized to nickel in personal objects. The hand dermatitis can then be provoked by the handling of nickel objects at work.
5. The dermatitis which originates primarily at work from chromate in cement or nickel in a nickel-plating bath can be maintained by involuntary contacts away from work. The dermatitis may thus continue even if the patient stops working.

A total of 80–90% of the occupationally caused dermatitis is localized on the hands. When a dermatitis starts on the body, it is rarely of occupational origin.

In earlier reports it has often been said that allergic contact dermatitis accounted for only 20% of all cases of occupational contact dermatitis. With increasing skill and interest in patch testing the relative incidence of the allergic type increases and is now estimated at 50% or more.

The relative incidence depends, of course, on the type of industrialization. In many countries chromate, rubber, epoxy and nickel predominate as occupational allergens.

Occupational dermatitis may occur in nearly all occupations but in some the risk is greater. The same causes, e.g. rubber gloves, are found in a number of occupations. This applies also to epoxy resin in the metal, plastic, construction, and ceramic industries.

A medical report on patients seen for compensation purposes should contain:

(1) Sources of information other than the patient (previous case notes, report from general practitioner, industrial medical officer, inspection of place of work)
(2) Family history of skin diseases, atopy, etc.
(3) Previous medical history. Skin diseases, especially in childhood
(4) Previous occupations
(5) Description of the work process
(6) Period in present occupation and in present employment
(7) Period of contact with assumed causal factors
(8) Other cases of dermatitis, and standard of hygiene at the place of work

(9) Time and site of initial skin complaints. Previous injury at the initial site
(10) Progress with approximate dates of gradual or sudden aggravation or improvement and the influence of holidays, weekends, etc.
(11) Degree of incapacity during period of illness. Dates of absence from work
(12) Therapy
(13) Clinical findings. Present state (Have the lesions been suppressed by topical steroids?)
(14) Special investigations: patch tests (positive and negative tests). Exposure tests. Examination for fungus
(15) Intercurrent diseases
(16) Diagnosis
(17) Common knowledge of risk at the occupation in question
(18) Conclusions (in terms understandable to nonmedical readers):
    (a) Probable connection between occupational activity and the present pathological condition, balanced against predisposing factors and contributory factors in spare time.
    (b) Possibility of continuing in present occupation. Necessity of rehabilitation
    (c) Probable prognosis.

13.1 Household dermatitis

A special form of "occupational dermatosis" takes the form of contact dermatitis induced by housework. Contact dermatitis on the hands caused by housework appears fairly common, probably the most common "occupational dermatosis". Detergents contribute to the origin of the irritant contact dermatitis. The wet work as such probably is as significant as the detergent itself. It must be taken into account, however, that many consumers use much too high concentrations of detergents and dishwashing liquids.

Rubber gloves are one of the causes. They themselves cause allergic dermatitis at the same time as they support the absorption of other substances which have already reached the skin. Common sensitizers are handlotions, spices, plants, nickel, topical medicaments for children and pets.

Contact urticaria is caused by fish, meat, lettuce and other vegetables, potatoes, fruits, and spices.

Those who do housework at home can seldom stop doing work which is bad for the hands. The dermatitis has a tendency to become chronic, but considerable prophylactic measures can be taken.

14. Irritants and sensitizers in occupations

Agriculture (farmers, animal handlers and keepers)

Irritants: Artificial fertilizers, disinfectants and cleansers for milking utensils, petrol, diesel oil.

Sensitizers: Rubber (boots, gloves, milking machines), cement, paints, local remedies for veterinary use, wood preservatives, plants, pesticides, antibiotics and preservatives in animal feed, (quindoxin, etho-xyquine), penicillin for mastitis, cobalt in animal feed.

Contact urticaria: Animal hair.

Artists

Irritants: Solvents, clay, plaster.

Sensitizers: Turpentine, cobalt, nickel and chromate in pigments, azo dyes, colophony, epoxy-, acrylic-, formaldehyde- resins.

Automobile mechanics

Irritants: Solvents, oils, cutting oils, paints, hand cleansers.

Sensitizers: Chromate (primers, anticorrosives, oils, welding fumes and cutting oils), nickel, cobalt, rubber, epoxy and acrylic resins, dipentene in thinners.

Baking and pastry-making

Irritants: Flour, detergents.

Sensitizers: Citrus fruits, flour improvers, thiamine, spices (cinnamon, cardamom), essential oils, food dyes.

Contact urticaria: Flour, essential oils.

Bartenders

Irritants: Detergents, citrus fruits.

Sensitizers: Flavouring agents.

Bathing attendants

Irritants: Detergents.
Sensitizers: Antimicrobial agents, formaldehyde, essential oils.

Bookbinders

Irritants: Glues, solvents, paper.
Sensitizers: Glues, formaldehyde, plastic monomers.

Building trade

Irritants: Cement, chalk, hydrochloric and hydrofluoric acids, glasswool, wood preservatives, organic tin compounds.
Sensitizers: Cement (chromate, cobalt), rubber and leather gloves, additives in shale oils, glues (phenol- or urea-formaldehyde resins), wood preservatives, teak, tar, epoxy resin, polyurethanes, rubber strip seals, joining material.

Butchers

Irritants: Detergents, meat, entrails.
Sensitizers: Nickel.
Contact   Animal tissues.
urticaria:

Canning industry

Irritants: Brine, syrup, prawns and shrimps.
Sensitizers: Asparagus, carrots, preservatives (hexamethylene tetramine in fish canning), rubber gloves.
Contact   Fruits, vegetables
urticaria:

Carpenters, cabinetmakers, timbermen

Irritants: French polish, solvents, glues, cleansers, wood preservatives, (also phototoxic). glassfiber.
Sensitizers: Exotic woods (teak, mahogany, rosewood, etc.), glues, polishes, turpentine, nickel, rubber (handles), colophony, epoxy-, acrylic-formaldehyde-, isocyanate-resins.

Chemical and pharmaceutical industry

Irritants and
Sensitizers: Numerous and specific for each working place.

Cleaning work

Irritants: Detergents, solvents.
Sensitizers: Rubber gloves, nickel, formaldehyde.

Coalminers

Irritants: Stone dust, coal dust, oil, grease, wood preservatives, cement, powdered limestone.

Sensitizers: Rubber (boots), face masks, explosives, chromate and cobalt in cement.

Cooks, catering industry

Irritants: Detergents, dressings, vinegar, fish, meat and vegetable juices.

Sensitizers: Vegetables (onions, garlic, lemons, lettuce, artichokes), knife handles (exotic woods), spices, formaldehyde.

Contact urticaria: Meat, fish, fruits, vegetables.

Dentists and dental technicians

Irritants: Soap, detergents, acrylic monomer, fluxes.

Sensitizers: Local anesthetics (tetracaine, procaine), mercury, rubber, UV-hardening acrylates, acrylic monomer, disinfectants (formaldehyde, eugenol), nickel, epoxy resin (filling), methylmethacrylate, periodontal dressing (balsam of Peru, colophony, eugenol), the catalyst methyl-p-toluenesulfonate in plastics used for sealing teeth.

Contact urticaria: Saliva.

Dyers

Irritants: Solvents, oxidizing and reducing agents, hypochlorite, hair removers.

Sensitizers: Dyes, chromate, formaldehyde.

Electricians

Irritants: Soldering flux.

Sensitizers: Soldering flux, insulating tape (rubber, resin, tar), rubber, nickel, bitumen, epoxy resins, glues (phenol-formaldehyde), polyurethanes.

Enamel workers

Irritants: Enamel powder.

Sensitizers: Chromate, nickel, cobalt.

Fishing

Irritants: Wet work, friction, oils, petrol, redfeed from mackerel.

Sensitizers: Tars, organic dyes in nets, rubber boots, rubber gloves.

Contact urticaria: Fish. "Aquatic irritant reactions" from toxins in sea organisms.

Floorlayers

Irritants: Solvents, detergents.

Sensitizers: Chromate (cement), epoxy resin, glues (phenol- and urea-formaldehyde), exotic woods, acrylates, varnish (urea-formaldehyde), polyurethanes.

Florists, gardeners, plant growers

Irritants: Manure, bulbs, fertilizers, pesticides.
Sensitizers: Plants (*Primula obconica*, chrysanthemum, tulips, narcissus, daffodils, alstromeria), formaldehyde, pesticides (e.g. thiuramsulfides), lichens (e.g. reindeer moss).

Food industry, foodhandler

Irritants: Detergents, vegetables.
Sensitizers: Rubber gloves, spices, vegetables, preservatives.
Contact   Vegetables, fruit, meat, fish.
urticaria:

Foundary work

Irritants: Oils, hand cleansers.
Sensitizers: Phenol- and carbamide-formaldehyde-, furan-, epoxy-resins, chromate (cement, gloves, bricks).

Glaziers

Sensitizers: Rubber, epoxy resin, joining material, exotic wood.

Hairdressers and barbers

Irritants: Shampoos, soaps, permanentwave liquids, bleaching agents.
Sensitizers: Hair and eyebrow dyes, rubber, nickel, perfumes.
Contact   Ammonium persulfate.
urticaria:

Histology technicians

Irritants: Solvents, formaldehyde.
Sensitizers: Formaldehyde, glutaraldehyde, organic dyes, acrylates.

Hospital personnel

Irritants: Disinfectants, quaternary ammonium compounds, hand creams, soaps, detergents.
Sensitizers: Rubber gloves, formaldehyde, antibacterial agents, piperazine, phenothiazines, hand creams, nickel, glutaraldehyde, acrylic monomer, nitrogen mustard, local anesthetics.

Household work

Irritants: Detergents, wet work, solvents, polishes, vegetables.

| Sensitizers: | Rubber (gloves), nickel, chromate, flowers and plants, turpentine (polishes), handcreams and lotions, handles of knives and irons, balsams, spices, citrus fruits. |
| Contact urticaria: | Vegetables, fruit, meat, fish, spices. |

Jewelers

| Irritants: | Solvents, fluxes. |
| Sensitizers: | Nickel, epoxy resins, enamels (chromate, nickel, cobalt). |

Laundry workers

| Irritants: | Detergents, bleaches, solvents. |
| Sensitizers: | Formaldehyde. |

Manicurists, beauticians

| Irritants: | Wet work. |
| Sensitizers: | Formaldehyde, cosmetics, acrylic monomers (nails), nail polish (sulfonamide-formaldehyde plastic), perfume. |

Masons

| Irritants: | Cement, chalk, bricks, acids. |
| Sensitizers: | Chromate and cobalt in cement, rubber and leather gloves, epoxy resin, exotic woods. |

Mechanics

| Irritants: | Solvents, detergents, degreasers, lubricants, oils, cooling system fluids, battery acid, soldering flux. |
| Sensitizers: | Rubber, chromate, nickel, epoxy resin. |

Metal workers

| Irritants: | Cutting and drilling oils, hand cleansers, solvents. |
| Sensitizers: | Nickel, chromate (antirust agents and dyes, welding fumes), cobalt, antibacterial agents and antioxidants in cutting oils. Chromate, cobalt, nickel may be found in cutting oil after it has been in use. |

Office workers

| Irritants: | Photocopy paper, NCR paper. |
| Sensitizers: | Rubber (erasing rubber, mats, cords, finger stalls), nickel (clips, scissors, typewriters), copying papers, glue, feltpen dyes. |

Painters

| Irritants: | Solvents, turpentine, thinner, paints, wallpaper adhesive, paint |

7

Sensitizers: Turpentine, thinner containing turpentine or dipentene (limonene), cobalt (dyes, driers), chromate (green, yellow), polyurethane-, epoxy-, acrylic-resins, glues (urea- and phenol-formaldehyde), varnish (colophony, urea-formaldehyde), preservatives in water-based paints and glues (e.g. chloracetamide, methylol-chloracetamide), putty (epoxy, acrylate, formaldehyde resins, polyurethane).

Photography

Irritants: Alkalis, reducing and oxidizing agents, solvents.
Sensitizers: Metol (p-aminophenol), color developers (azo compounds), chromate, formaldehyde.

Plastics industry

Irritants: Solvents, styrene, oxidizing agents, acids.
Sensitizers: Low molecular raw material, hardeners, additives, dyes.

Platers

Irritants: Solvents, paints.
Sensitizers: Chromate in paints and on zinc galvanized sheets, glues.

Plating industry, electroplating

Irritants: Metal cleaners, alkalis, acids, detergents, heat, dust from metal blasting.
Sensitizers: Chromate, nickel, cobalt, gold, mercury, rubber gloves, glanzing agents.

Plumbers

Irritants: Oils, hand cleansers, soldering flux.
Sensitizers: Rubber (gloves, packings, tubes), nickel, chromate (cement, antirust paint), glues, hydrazine.

Printers

Irritants: Solvents.
Sensitizers: Nickel, chromate, cobalt, colophony, paper finishes, glues, turpentine, azo dyes, formaldehyde, printing plates (acrylates and other chemicals), UV-hardening acrylates in printing ink, rubber gloves.

Radio, television electronic repairmen

Irritants: Soldering flux.
Sensitizers: Soldering flux (hydrazine), epoxy resin, colophony (soldering), nickel, chromate.

Restaurant personnel

Irritants: Detergents, vegetables, citrus fruits, shrimps, herring.
Sensitizers: Nickel, spices, vegetables, exotic wood (knife handle).
Contact   Vegetables, fruit, meat, fish.
urticaria:

Road workers

Irritants: Sand/oil mixture, hand cleansers, asphalt (phototoxic).
Sensitizers: Cement, gloves (leather, rubber), epoxy resin, tar, chromate in antirust paint.

Rubber workers

Irritants: Talcum, zinc stearate, solvents.
Sensitizers: Rubber chemicals, organic dyes, tars, colophony, chromate, cobalt, phenol-formaldehyde resin.

Shoemakers

Irritants: Solvents.
Sensitizers: Leather (formaldehyde, chromate, dyes), rubber, colophony, glues (e.g. p-tert. butylphenol-formaldehyde).

Shop assistants

Irritants: Detergents, vegetables, fruit, meat, fish.
Sensitizers: Nickel.
Contact   Fruits, vegetables.
urticaria:

Tanners

Irritants: Acids, alkalis, reducing and oxidizing agents.
Sensitizers: Chromate, formaldehyde, vegetable tanning agents, glutaraldehyde, finishes, antimildew agents, dyes, resins.

Textile workers

Irritants: Solvents, bleaching agents, fibers.
Sensitizers: Finishes (formaldehyde resins), dyes, mordants, nickel, diazo paper.

Veterinarians

Irritants: Hypochlorite, quaternary ammonium compounds, cresol, rectal and vaginal examination of cattle.
Sensitizers: Rubber gloves, antibiotics (penicillin, streptomycin, neomycin, tylosine tartrate, virginiamycin), antimycotic agents, MBT in

medicaments. (Tuberculin for injection in animals can elicit reactions on the hands).

Contact urticaria: Animal hair and dander, cow placenta, animal tissues.

Welders

Irritants: Oil.
Sensitizers: Chromate (welding fumes, gloves), nickel, cobalt.

Woodworkers

Sensitizers: Woods, colophony, turpentine, balsams, tars, lacquers, Frullania, lichens, glues, wood preservatives.

15. Predisposing factors

Only people with certain susceptibility to irritants seem to develop irritant contact dermatitis of chronic type, and then often from rather mild irritants. Most people may have contact with irritants for years without developing this type of dermatitis. The susceptibility cannot be predicted. People with atopic constitution or otherwise dry skin possibly develop irritant dermatitis more easily than others. Yet irritant contact dermatitis of acute type may be developed in most people from sufficient exposure.

It is not known why some people develop contact allergy more easily than others. It is genetically related, but a connecting factor may also be an increased inherent penetrability of the skin.

There are controversial opinions as to whether there is any difference in the inherent capacity between the sexes to develop irritant or allergic dermatitis. Some investigations indicate that women more easily develop delayed contact allergy. However, contact with allergens differs for the two sexes. Women are more exposed to contact with nickel and men to chromate. During pregnancy the skin appears more easily damaged by irritant factors. Allergy reactivity declines with age, but susceptibility to irritants increases.

A person once allergic to one substance and having a chronic or relapsing dermatitis more easily develops sensitivity to new substances, e.g. cosmetics, rubber gloves and topical medicaments. This might be due to increased absorption in the damaged skin. Also irritant reactions facilitate sensitization.

The time of the year plays a role. During hot summers increased sweating can cause an increased provocation of the contact allergy from clothes, as from objects carried in the hands. During the winter when the relative humidity is reduced indoors, skin dryness appears. This leads to cracks forming pathways for irritants and allergens.

Heavy palmar sweating predisposes to dermatitis caused by released chromium compounds in leather gloves and dyes in textile gloves. Sweating on the soles means that rubber, tanning material, dyes, etc., in socks, stockings and shoes are more easily released. Sweating in the axillae causes release of dyes from clothes.

If personal hygiene is poor – lacking in care of the body and clothes but also neglect of protective material – contact with substances damaging to the skin is increased. It is important how the skin is cared for. If an emollient is applied after work, dryness and cracks do not develop so easily.

16. Systematic examination of contact dermatitis

16.1 Preliminary history

From the history and examination findings provisional diagnosis is made. It should be observed that contact dermatitis may develop secondarily to another type of dermatitis. Contact allergy should always be suspected when the dermatitis is localized on the hands. Sometimes a quickly taken history can give clear information about the origin. That is especially so with allergic contact dermatitis with typical localization. But often a careful history is needed.

16.2 History

A carefully compiled history requires considerable time and should be supplemented through return visits.

16.3 Family history

Dermatitis in relatives especially during childhood can mean that the patient too is predisposed to atopic dermatitis.

16.4 Illnesses of the patient in childhood

Dermatitis or asthma in the history may indicate an atopic constitution.

16.5 Localization

This especielly means the initial localization, e.g. feet, leg wound, ring finger, injury site, under jewelry or watch.

16.6 Progress of the illness

The localization of the dermatitis at onset can give information as to a possible allergen. A primary injury may facilitate the development of dermatitis through secondary infection or through sensitizing to topical medicaments including adhesive tape. Strong itching, angry erythema, small vesicles and quick alterations speak for the contact allergic nature of the dermatitis. Considerable improvement on weekends, holidays or short sick leaves and swift worsening when returned to work suggests contact dermatitis of allergic nature and that the allergen is present at the place of work. A slow worsening over some weeks on return after sick leave suggests and irritant type.

16.7 Occupational activity

Work for a long time in the same occupation and even in the same job does not prevent the cause of the contact dermatitis from being present in the work. It can take decades before sensitization takes place.

Irritant contact dermatitis may develop slowly but an injury or local infection may cause a relatively quick emergence. The work history must be detailed as regards contacts which take place at intervals of several weeks. Cleansers and protective equipment, e.g. rubber gloves, can amount to an injurious contact. When necessary, information should be obtained from the employers.

16.8 Hobbies

Not infrequently the cause of the contact dermatitis is found in a hobby, such as painting, carpentry, pasting, cementing, gluing, sewing, weaving, photographic developing, enamel work and other types of "do-it-yourself" and sports.

16.9 Chemical-technical substances

Cleansers, solvents, polishes, shoe polish, mothballs, etc., which are found in the home can cause irritant and allergic contact dermatitis.

102

16.10 Plants

In all contact dermatitis on the hands, forearms and face, plants should be suspected. Orange peel can, through its irritant effect, maintain a contact dermatitis on the hands.

16.11 Topical treatment and cosmetics

Topical treatment prescribed by a doctor and that started by the patient himself can cause contact allergy secondarily. Application of topical medicaments on other family members, pets and cattle can cause hand dermatitis.

16.12 Connubial or "consort" contactants

Substances inducing sensitivity or eliciting dermatitis may be transmitted from partners: perfumes, deodorants, hairdyes, lipsticks, lanolin/propyleneglycol/preservatives in creams and vaginal lubricants, perfumes or disinfectants in feminine hygiene sprays or sanitary napkins, contraceptive agents, antifungals, benzoylperoxide in acne medicaments, rubber chemicals in condoms. Sensitizing compounds might also be brought home on skin or on clothing from work. Irritants, for example fiberglass, might be transmitted directly or via washing machines. Seminal fluid can cause contact urticaria or generalized itching, urticaria and an anaphylactoid response in the female.

16.13 Appearance of dermatitis

Papules, vesicles, point-shaped discharge and swelling point most closely to allergic contact dermatitis but may also be present in irritant contact dermatitis. Dryness and cracks indicate irritant reaction but may also be present in allergic dermatitis when the lesions have been present for a while. Sore cracks and swelling over the finger joints and crusty discharge indicate secondary infection.

16.14 Appearance of normal skin

Note signs of pronounced fatty or dry skin, seborrhoeic, psoriatic or atopic lesions. The whole body should be examined. In hand dermatitis, the feet must always be inspected for fungal infection or dermatitis from antifungal medicaments.

16.15 Patch testing

In exceptional cases it is sufficient to patch test with the substance which is the likely cause. In many cases, however, there is contact allergy to several substances at the same time. In all cases where the cause is not clear and especially when the patient does not recover quickly after the suspected contact allergen has been removed, patch testing should be performed with standard substances and with suspected substances according to the information from the case history. Completely negative results often lead to the diagnosis of irritant contact dermatitis, but it should not be forgotten that it is difficult to obtain information about all contacts the patient has had and that the testing technique still suffers from serious shortcomings.

16.16 Chemical analysis

Tracing formaldehyde and nickel in contactants with simple methods can give valuable information (see 4.6 and 4.8.2).

16.17 Link between history, status and patch test result

Such a link must be carefully examined. Thus, a positive test result can be unrelated to the existing contact dermatitis. We should remember that the details of the occurrence of the standard test substances are not yet known. An actual link between case history, status and test reactions should lead to adequate treatment. However, we must realize that we fail to establish the right diagnosis or trace the cause in maybe 20–30% of cases examined.

17. Prevention

This chapter is concerned with *primary prevention,* i.e. inhibition of onset of contact dermatitis. *Secondary prevention*-inhibition of relapses- and *tertiary prevention*-inhibition of worsening- are parts of treatment. Many different factors contribute to the origin of contact dermatitis and these can probably never be completely preventable. Often it is impossible, for practical reasons, for individuals completely to follow the protective rules at work. It is not sufficient to make protective rules and to inform staff; one must see that they are complied with. There has been most success in industries with industrial medical officers and safety engineers.

Information on the potential risks to workers and supervisors is important. It is most efficient if it is done before the starting of a new process.

Workers handling hazardous chemicals, for example epoxy resin systems, should be specially trained.

Preemployment patch testing with potential sensitizers should not be performed. A careful history of new employees is of great value and patch testing should be performed if previous dermatitis has not been properly examined. The occurrence of contact dermatitis can be hindered to a certain extent by avoiding the employment of people with atopic dermatitis in work which is particularly traumatizing. This is especially so with work involving moisture or solvents.

All chemicals at a work site should be listed. Industrial data sheets should be present. All packages of chemicals used at a site should be labeled about the content and precautions. If there are prescriptions by legislation they should be present at the work site. When new chemicals are suggested to be used, predictive test results on irritant capacity and allergenicity should be considered.

Good housekeeping is important. Chemicals, tools and protective materials should be kept in place and as clean as possible.

Often personal protectives such as gloves, aprons, boots, glasses and masks are necessary. Gloves should be plastic and not rubber when possible. Many substances, particularly when dissolved in organic solvents, penetrate plastic and rubber gloves within 1/2 hour. The penetration continues when the gloves are not in use. When the lining is chemically contaminated, the gloves can be more dangerous than no gloves at all because of increased penetration with occlusion.

Hygiene plays the most important role. If chemicals remain on the skin for 24 hours instead of 8 hours, sensitization and irritation occur more easily. Remove chemicals as quickly and as completely as possible. When forced to use skin-damaging substances, irritants or allergens, protect the skin as far as possible from contact. This can be done with automation. Not infrequently chemicals are transferred with scoops whereby they contaminate the working area around them. Use closed systems with hoses and taps instead.

Dusty chemicals, e.g. alkalies, detergents, enzymes, dyes, should be used as "masterbatches". That means that the chemicals are blended with small portions of the main material, e.g. dyes in plastic and rubber chemicals in rubber. Dishwasher detergents in powder form raise a dust adhering to the skin and are more irritating than corresponding liquids.

Among epoxy hardeners, adducts and polyaminoamides free from aliphatic amines are recommended.

The sensitizing chromate in cement can be "eliminated" by addition of iron sulfate to the cement/sand/water mixture (0.3% calculated to the cement content).

Attempts have been made to remove certain irritants or strong sensitizers. In several countries the use of p-phenylenediamine in hair dyes has been forbidden. In several countries cosmetics and drugs must go through special testing. Acetylated lanolin is considered to be less allergenic than lanolin. The outbreaks of dermatitis from halogenated salicylanilides should have been avoidable. Dichromate sulfuric acid for cleaning of laboratory glassware can be replaced by detergents. Chromate and hydrazine as anticorrosive agents in cooling water can be replaced by other agents. Primula dermatitis in Europe could be abolished almost completely by legal means. Nickel dermatitis from suspenders has decreased through the use of tights, but neither should other personal objects be made of nickel. Diesel oil should not be part of molding oil in cement casting. Hand cleansers containing alkali, aromatic solvents or perfume can be replaced. For the most part, however, it is impossible to replace many chemicals, as they are necessary to the industrial process, e.g. cement and epoxy resin.

Other chemicals are now, for technical reasons, used less than before. Thus it is unusual to see the strongly sensitizing turpentine. It has been replaced by other nonsensitizing solvents such as white spirit (kerosene) and thinner.

It is important that causes of contact dermatitis are investigated in detail, especially those of allergic contact dermatitis. In that way the risks in a work site can be discovered. And new substances in, e.g. resins, rubber, cosmetics, medicaments, and clothes can be traced.

In treatment of minor injuries in industry often unnecessary ointments are used which contain sensitizing substances, e.g. local anesthetics.

In the home much can be done to prevent the occurrence of contact dermatitis. However, for practical reasons, an information campaign is difficult. Protective measures can be proposed only after the occurrence of a contact dermatitis. Much could be gained, however, if plastic gloves were used instead of rubber gloves. Washing machines, dishwashers, and long-handled brushes have great importance. Detergents and other cleansers should be used in the concentrations suggested by the manufacturers. In the long run much can be done by the community for prevention of contact dermatitis both in the occupational and the nonoccupational environment.

17.1 Skin cleansing

For prevention of contact dermatitis it is important that suitable methods are used for skin cleansing. This is especially so in industry. The choice of cleanser is determined by the type of dirt and its solubility. At the same work site several types of cleansers may be necessary. The most effective should not be used by everyone! It often happens that workmen use solvents which are available at work for other purposes, but this is undesirable.

The cleanser which is least irritating is soap and water. For most occasions this is sufficient, but if it is not, soap powder can be mixed with sawdust. Sand, quartz and pumice stone are unsuitable as they scratch the skin surface.

Sometimes, detergents, e.g. alkylaryl sulfonate and alkylether sulfate, are necessary, but they involve a certain amount of risk to the skin, especially if they are used in high concentrations.

For special dirt, certain oils, plastics, tars, etc., "water-free cleansing cream" is used. There are different types of these for different types of dirt. The cream is rubbed into the skin and the dirt is wiped off with paper towels. The creams contain solvents, but these should not contain aromatics, since the latter more easily irritate the skin. The addition of strong alkalis is extremely unsuitable.

In many jobs barrier creams are suitable. They should be adapted to the type of dirt. Commonly they do not prevent penetration by the injurious substances but are important because the dirt can more easily be washed away with a milder cleanser.

The skin should be well dried after washing. If paper towels are used, they should not be of too hard a paper. Drying in a stream of air is often unsuitable as the skin then easily gets dried out.

An unscented cream should be rubbed on the hands after washing to minimize drying.

Especially in dusty occupations showers should be taken regularly every day. The hair should be washed so that any allergens are removed.

Principles of prevention

At the work site
Information of workers and supervisors
Training of workers in special processes
Preemployment examination
List of chemicals
Labeling of chemicals
Judging of potential hazards of new chemicals
Good housekeeping
Personal protection
Personal hygiene
Proper handcleaning agents
Barrier creams
Automation
Replacement of chemicals
Modification of chemicals
Tracing of causes of skin diseases
Proper treatment of injuries

In the community
Research
Application of research results
Legislation
Departments of occupational dermatology
Vocational guidance
Predictive testing
Replacement of chemicals
Change of chemical properties

18. Treatment

The patient should be carefully informed about the causes of his contact dermatitis, which usually means a detailed investigation. In allergic contact dermatitis all products containing the actual allergen must be listed. The information should include substances involved in cross-sensitivity. If there are many such substances, e.g. as in allergy to balsams, nickel, chromate, rubber, the patient should be given a list.

It is important to have the patient's cooperation. At each return visit the presence of the allergen and the patient's attempts to eliminate it should be discussed. This is especially important when the dermatitis is localized on the hand.

It is important that the patient is informed that the allergy remains even when the dermatitis is healed and that the risk of recurrence on renewed contact may persist for the rest of his life.

Mention – especially when dealing with hand dermatitis – that the tolerance of injurious substances is reduced for several months after the skin looks healed to the naked eye. For this reason, a warning should be given against detergents, dishwashing liquids, hair shampoo, solvents, etc.

Topical treatment with corticoids is used to stop eczematous inflammation. This applies to the allergic and the irritant type. The corticoids do not themselves influence the allergic process but only the inflammation.

High potency corticoids should not be used for long periods because of a risk of skin atrophy. Treatment with hydrocortisone or low potency steroids can continue for years. Hand dermatitis in, e.g. brick-layers with chromate allergy should be treated in this way, which often means that continued work in the same occupation will be possible. The corticoid treatment should be gradually withdrawn and replaced by an indifferent ointment, e.g. unperfumed cold cream. It should be pointed out that ointments and creams of indifferent type cannot be applied to weeping dermatitis, although corticoid creams can be. If the corticoids are used locally in the form of liniment or spray, drying of the skin may easily occur. Tar is usually avoided as it is cosmetically unsatisfactory and is sensitizing and phototoxic.

Elimination of the allergen can sometimes be done by means of special measures.

Organic dyes in hair which have caused dermatitis can be removed by repeated washing with common salt 15% and hydrogen peroxide 1% in water.

In nickel allergy as many nickel objects as possible should be removed. They can most suitably be replaced by plastic. Those that cannot be removed should be painted over with colorless metal lacquer. Pockets in which loose keys or coins have been kept should be replaced. Nickel should be traced in the environment by help of a simple stick test (see Nickel 4.8.2) Patients sensitized to nickel objects should be warned not to expose the hands to strong irritants. Nickel hand dermatitis often starts after such an exposure that increases the absorption of nickel.

In dermatitis caused by chromate allergy a common contact source is matches; the patient should avoid using them. Pockets where matches were kept should be turned inside out and thoroughly brushed.

Patients with ring dermatitis and negative patch tests should be warned not to expose the hands to strong irritants, as the ring dermatitis might be the first sign of irritant contact dermatitis.

Eyeglass frames can be coated with polyurethane varnish.

Hyposensitization usually has no effect in cases of contact allergy.

Systematic treatment with corticoids should be given only in serious contact allergy. In case of extreme swelling of the face, e.g. caused by plant allergy, however, such treatment can be given for quick relief. When systematic corticoid treatment is started, the treatment should continue for some weeks while the skin becomes free of the allergen. Otherwise exacerbation cannot be avoided.

Systemic antibiotic treatment is often appropriate. For example, contact dermatitis on the hands may be maintained by a secondary infection, which appears as tender red cracks or swelling of the fingers, especially at the joints. Large pustules on the hands point to infection with beta-streptococci. Locally applied antibacterial agents incorporated in corticosteroid preparations have limited effect.

Antihistamines should never be used topically as they are in general strong sensitizers. Antihistamines given orally can sometimes relieve a profound itch and may then best be given in the evening for their sedative properties.

Acute treatment
Small burns should be treated with an antibacterial agent under thin sterile dressing.

Caustic injuries from alkalis or acids should first be thoroughly rinsed under running cold water for at least 30 minutes, preferably for 1 hour. The treatment with water should start immediately. It is not advantageous to apply neutralizing agents.

Hot pitch or resins should be flushed with cold water and left in place.

Dry calcium oxide, quicklime, should be removed from the skin as much as possible before flushing with water.

Oxalic acid should be removed by water and the skin then treated with calcium or magnesium salts.

If the caustic effect has been caused by bromine or iodine, the skin surface should be treated with 5% sodium thiosulfate solution; if caused by yellow phosphorus it should be washed with 1% copper sulfate solution. After contact with phenols and chlorophenols the damage is washed with water and then with polyethyleneglycol 400 or 10% alcohol.

Chemical burn from hydrofluoric acid should be treated with water and then with 2.5% calcium gluconate in a jelly (e.g. hydrated hydroxy methylcellulose). Sometimes injection of 10% calcium gluconate in the lesion may be made. No local anesthetics should be applied. Disappearance of pain is a sign of successful treatment with calcium gluconate.

All bullae should be completely evacuated as they may contain chemicals giving local or systemic injury, e.g. organic mercury compounds.

Chemical burns with necrosis from hydrofluoric acid, cement or other chemicals should preferably be removed by surgical excision in acute phase. The healing time may then be decreased from 2–3 months to 3–4 weeks.

Reactions to animal toxins should be treated with as hot water as tolerated.

18.1 Instructions for patients

In cases of hand dermatitis it is especially useful to give the patient written instructions on general irritants and special allergens. Here are some examples:

You are allergic to CHROMIUM

The allergy is going to remain many years after the dermatitis has healed. To facilitate healing and prevent relapse, you should avoid contact with the following:

Leather: e.g. in gloves, shoe leather, pet leashes.

Cement: Concrete that has set, however, is not dangerous.

Matches: should not be kept in the pocket. The pockets should be brushed clean if matches have previously been kept in them. Use a cigarette lighter.

Anticorrosive paint: Yellow and red paint for rust protection on metal.

Welding fumes.

Lithographic chemicals.

Zinc galvanized iron sheets.

Green baize: On gaming and billiard tables.

Ashes: Especially from wood and rubbish.

Hand Dermatitis

To speed healing and prevent relapse of your dermatitis you should remember.

1. *Hand washing.* Use lukewarm water and soap without any perfume, tar or sulfur. The soap should be used sparingly and the hands rinsed thoroughly. Dry carefully with a clean towel, not forgetting to dry between the fingers.
2. As far as possible avoid direct contact with *detergents* and other strong cleansing agents. Measure the quantity according to the maker's directions, otherwise they

may be too strong. Keep the packages clean to avoid irritation from detergent on the outside.

3. Avoid direct contact with *shampoo*. Let somebody else shampoo your hair, or use plastic gloves.

4. Avoid direct contact with *metal polish, wax polish, shoe, floor, car, furniture, and window polishes.*

5. Be careful not to get *solvents* such as white spirit, petrol, kerosene, acetone, trichlorethylene, turpentine and thinners, on the skin.

6. Don't peel or squeeze *oranges, lemons* or *grapefruit* with bare hands.

7. Don't apply *hair lotion, hair cream* or *hair dye* with bare hands.

8. Wear gloves in cold weather.

9. *Rings* should not be worn during housework or other work, even when the dermatitis has healed. Rings should be cleaned frequently on the inside with a brush, and left in ammonia water overnight, then rinsed thoroughly. Never wash your hands with soap when wearing a ring.

10. For dishwashing, use running water if possible.

11. If *gloves* are used for washing dishes and clothes they should be *plastic* and not rubber, since the latter often cause dermatitis. They should not be worn for more than 15–20 min at a time. If water happens to enter a glove, it must immediately be taken off. Rinse them under the hot water tap several times a week. They should be worn only a few times before they are washed. Buy several pair of plastic gloves at a time. Use preferably disposable gloves.

12. Try to work as carefully as possible. Do not spread chemicals in your

13. *Remember that the resistance of the skin is lowered for at least 4 or 5 months after the dermatitis appears to be completely healed, so continue to follow the instructions.*

14. Washing machines and dishwashers may help to prevent further attacks.

19. Rehabilitation

The aim of rehabilitation is to bring the patient back to the best possible health and optimal activity and adjustment to the surrounding world. This means both a medical and a social goal. Rehabilitation is relevant to all types of disease no matter whether they are occupational or not.

In cases of contact dermatitis there is an imperative need for the cause of the dermatitis to be investigated in detail. This applies to causes both at the place of work and in the leisure time environment, including personal belongings.

Bring the patient back to his old place of work, if possible. Relapse of dermatitis when the patient returns to his place of work after sick leave should not be an absolute indication for change of worksite. Numerous contact allergens can be removed, e.g. rubber and leather gloves, rubber handles, hand balsams. Strong hand cleansers can be exchanged for milder ones.

Personal prophylaxis in the form of plastic gloves, aprons, etc., may sometimes give enough protection. It is possible to bring most building workers and bricklayers back to their old work, in spite of their having contact allergy to chromate in cement, by avoiding contacts of other chromium compounds and undergoing continuous hydrocortisone treatment. The patient should be informed that change of work does not guarantee complete healing. About 75% of these patients can continue in their jobs. When the contact allergens are present as dust or vapor which cannot be removed (e.g. teak, epoxy compounds), it is usually impossible to continue in the same work if processing cannot be stopped in the working area. Contact allergy to *Chrysanthemum* usually makes work change necessary.

People with atopic dermatitis usually cannot continue to work with irritants, particularly if they have had hand dermatitis also previously.

Irritant contact dermatitis of chronic type often leads to change of work, but irritant dermatitis of acute type, for example from hairdressing or cutting oil does not necessarily do so.

In the case of dermatitis from work at home special problems arise. These patients for natural reasons, cannot generally be off sick for long enough to allow the dermatitis time to heal properly. Many contact allergens (rubber gloves, plants, handlotion, spices, nickel handles, etc.) can be removed.

If change of work with or without retraining is necessary, it is of the greatest importance that choice of the new place of work is the right one. If the dermatitis is on the hands, whatever the original cause, the new work must not involve contact with irritants.

Proper rehabilitation involves not only medical but also social activities, e.g. by employer, welfare officer, insurance company, social institutions, labor inspectors and trade union. However, these contributions depend much on the legislation in the country. Many social and personnel factors are often more decisive for change of work than the medical problems.

Physicians should always be aware that the medical task is to give advice based on facts, but not to ultimately decide a patient's future.

20. Prognosis

Our knowledge of prognosis in contact dermatitis is incomplete. Factors which influence the prognosis are the cause of the contact dermatitis, how long a time elapses before adequate treatment is begun, and whether the patient has been informed of where the provoking factors occur and thereby has a chance to avoid them.

Short periods of contact dermatitis from plants and cosmetics are common. The cause in many cases is obvious and the dermatitis does not often require medical examination. Nickel contact dermatitis from personal objects is common and the connection easy to find. About 10% of adult women are allergic to nickel but less than half of them experience any problem when they have removed the objects.

Allergic contact dermatitis to such industrial chemicals as are used in restricted places and are not present in the leisure time environment or personal belongings has a good prognosis. Allergic dermatitis caused by chromate and nickel has a poor prognosis since those substances are present to such a large extent in our everyday life.

Irritant contact dermatitis on the hands also has a bad prognosis, since the constitutional factor is so decisive. Irritant reactions of acute type usually have a good prognosis. Several workers get irritant reactions in ordinary jobs after a long period of holidays. The dermatitis clears up spontaneously when the skin get "hardened".

Leg eczema can improve quickly if medicaments which caused secondary allergic contact dermatitis are removed.

Slow healing depends upon several different factors. A secondary infection, e.g. on the hands, can produce slight symptoms and be overlooked, but can maintain the contact dermatitis for a long time. If the patient exposes himself to irritants or does not eliminate the allergens, the healing is hindered. However, even during treatment, there may have been a sensitization to e.g. topical treatment preparations. In this respect special attention should be paid to local antibiotics, vehicles, preservatives and corticosteroids. Sensitization to these substances may occur even when they are part of a corticosteroid treatment and the corticosteroid effect can thereby "hide" the contact allergy. Secondary sensitization to nickel, balsams and rubber occurs. To determine whether such sensitization has taken place, repeated patch testing may become necessary. Sometimes the patient does not follow the instructions about the treatment.

When there is a slow healing, the contact dermatitis diagnosis should be taken under new consideration.

Several patients who change jobs do not clear up completely, yet they have to change as they would not have been able to work at all in their original jobs.

Most common causes of chronicity of contact dermatitis
Wrong diagnoses – often hand psoriasis
Ubiquitous allergens
Unknown source of the allergen
Unknown allergy
Cross allergens
Sensitization to the medicament used
Photosensitivity
No treatment at home
Maltreatment of the skin
Irritant at home or in hobby work
Infection
Strong endogenous factors

References

Adams, R. M.: *Occupational Contact Dermatitis*. J. B. Lippincott Co., Philadelphia, 1969.

van Alphen, J.: *Rubber Chemicals*. Elsevier Publ. Co., Amsterdam, 1979.

Bandmann H.-J. & Dohn, W.: *Die Epicutantestung*. Verlag J. F. Bergmann, München, 1967.

Bandmann, H.-J. & Dohn, W.: *Patch Testing*. Springer-Verlag 1973.

Bandmann, H.-J. & Fregert, S.: *Epicutantestung*. Springer-Verlag, Berlin, Heidelberg, New York, 1973.

Calman, C. D., editor: *Contact Dermatitis*. Environmental and Occupational Dermatitis, Issues bimonthly from 1975, Munksgaard, DK–1016 Copenhagen.

Colour Index (1971–1975) The society of Dyes and Colourists and the American Association of Textile Chemists and Colorists.

Cromin, E.: *Contact Dermatitis*. Chunchill Livingstone, Edinburgh, 1980.

Ducombes, G. & Chabeau, G.: *Dermato-allergologie de Contact*. Masson, 1979.

Fisher, A. A.: *Contact Dermatitis*. Lea & Febiger, Philadelphia, 1973.

Foussereau, J. & Benezra, C.: *Les Eczémas Allergiques Professionnels*. Masson & Cie, Paris, 1970. (English ed., 1980).

Fregert, S. & Bandmann, H.-J.: *Patch Testing*. Springer-Verlag, Berlin, Heidelberg, New York, 1975.

Handbook of Chemistry and Physics, Technical Rubber Co., Cleveland 1978–1979.

Hjorth, N. & Fregert, S.: Contact Dermatitis In *Textbook of Dermatology*. Ed.: Rook, A., Wilkinson, D. S. & Ebling, F. J. G. Blackwell Scient. Publ., Oxford, 3rd ed., 1979.

Magnusson, B. & Kligman, A. M.. Allergic contact dermatitis in the guinea pig. Identification of contact allergens. C. C. Thomas Publisher, Springfield, III, 1956.

Malten, K. E. & Zielhuis, R. L.: *Industrial Toxicology and Dermatology in the Production and Progressing of Plastics*. Elsevier Publ. Co., Amsterdam, London, New York, 1964.

Malten, K. E., Nater, J.-P. & van Ketel, W. G.: *Patch Testing Guidelines*. Dekker & van de Vegt, Nijmegen, 1976.

Marzulli, F. N. & Maibach, H. I., Ed.: Dermatotoxicology and pharmacology. In *Advances in Modern Toxicology*, Vol. 4, 1977, Hemisphere Publ. Corp., John Wiley & Sons.

Mitchel, J. & Rook, A.: *Botanical Dermatology*. Plants injurious to the skin. Greengrass Ltd., 691W, 28 Ave. Vancouver, Canada V5Z 2H4.

Merck Index, An Encyclopedia of Chemicals and Drugs. Merck & Co., Rahway, U. S.

Norman, F. E. editor: CTFA Cosmetic Ingredient Dictionary. The Cosmetic, Toiletry and Fragrance Association, Inc., Washington D. C., 1977.

Lachapelle, J. M.: *Dermatoses Professionnelles*. Clinique-diagnostic-prevention-legislation, Fonteyn Medical Books, Louvain, Belgium, 1978.

Sax, N. J., editor: Dangerous properties of industrial materials, Van Nostrand Reinhold Co., N Y, 1979.

Wilkinson, D. S., Fregert, S., Magnusson, B., Bandmann, H.-J., Calnan, C. D., Cronin, E., Hjorth, N., Maibach, H. J., Malten, K. E., Meneghini, C. L., Pirilä, V.:Terminology of contact dermatitis. *Acta Derm.-venereol.* **50**, 2871, 1970.

22. Test substances

Test substances proposed by the ICDRG are available from TROLAB, 6B Hansens Allé, DK-2900 Hellerup, Denmark.

22.1 ICDRG standard test series

1. Potassium dichromate, 0.5% petrolatum
2. p-Phenylenediamine, 1% petrolatum
3. Thiuram rubber mixture, petrolatum[1]
4. Neomycin, 20% petrolatum
5. Cobalt chloride, 1% petrolatum
6. Caine mixture, petrolatum[2]
7. Nickel sulfate, 2.5% petrolatum
8. Chinoform, 5% petrolatum
9. Colophony (rosin), 20% petrolatum
10. Parabens, petrolatum[3]
11. PPD rubber mixture, petrolatum[4]
12. Wool alcohols, 30% petrolatum
13. MBT rubber mixture, petrolatum[5]
14. Epoxy resin, 1% petrolatum
15. Balsam of Peru, 25% petrolatum
16. p-tert. Butyl-formaldehyde resin, 1% petrolatum
17. Carba rubber mixture[6]
18. Formaldehyde, 2% water
19. Ethylenediamine-HCl, 1% petrolatum
20. Perfume mixture[7], 2% each, petrolatum

---

[1] Tetramethylthiuram-disulfide (TMTD), 0.25%
Tetramethylthiuram-monosulfide (TMTM), 0.25%
Tetraethylthiuram-disulfide (TETD), 0.25%
Dipenthamethylenethiuram-disulfide (PTD), 0.25%

[2] Cinchocaine, 1%. Amethocaine, 1%. Cyclomethycaine, 1%. Benzocaine, 5%

[3] Methyl-, ethyl-, propyl-, butyl-, benzyl-p-hydroxy-benzoates, 3% each
[4] Phenyl-cyclo-hexyl-para-phenylenediamine (CPPD), 0.25%
   Phenyl-iso-propyl-para-phenylenediamine (IPPD), 0.10%
   Diphenyl-para-phenylenediamine (DPPD), 0.25%
[5] Mercaptobenzothiazole (MBT), 0.25%
   N-cyclo-hexyl-benzothiazyl-sulphenamide (CBS), 0.25%
   Di-beta-naphthyl-para-phenylenediamine (DBNPD), 0.5%
   Morpholinyl-mercaptobenzothiazole (MOR), 0.25%
[6] Diphenylguanidine (DPG), 1%
   bis(Diethyldithiocarbamate)zinc (ZDC), 1%
   bis(Dibutyldithiocarbamate)zinc (ZBC), 1%
[7] Amyl cinnamic aldehyde
   Cinnamic aldehyde
   Cinnamic alcohol
   Oak moss absolute
   Hydroxycitronellal
   Eugenol
   Isoeugenol
   Geraniol

22.2 NACDG standard series

Benzyl alcohol, 5%
Potassium dichromate, 0.5%
Wool alcohol, 30%
Mercaptobenzthiazole, 1%
Neomycin sulfate, 20%
Ethylenediamine-diHCl, 1%
Quaternium 15, 2%
Imidazolidinyl urea, 2%
Ammoniated mercury, 1%
Paraben mixture*
Formaldehyde, 2%
Carba rubber mixture**
Paraphenylenediamine, 1%
Lanolin, 100%
Thiuram rubber mixture**
Mercapto rubber mixture**
Caine mixture**
Epoxy resin, 1%
p-Chloro-m-xylenol, 1%
Black rubber mixture**
p-tert-Butylphenol-formaldehyde resin, 2%

Perfume mixture**

. . . .

Nickel sulfate, 2.5% (optional to be applied simultaneously or separately)

* Methyl-, ethyl-, propyl-, butyl-, p-hydroxybenzoates, 3% each

** See 22.1

22.3 Additional test chemicals

Vehicles: pet. is the equivalent of yellow soft paraffin. B.P., and petrolatum U.S.P. MEK is methyl ethylketone. O.O. is olive oil, acet. is acetone, alc. is ethanol.

Abietic acid, 5% pet.
Abietic alcohol, 5% pet.
Acrylate monomers, 0.1–5% pet.
Acrylates UV-hardening,
  0.05–0.1% pet.
Acrylic acid, 0.1% pet.
Acrylonitrile, 1% pet.
Alantolactone (Helenin), 0.1% pet.
Alcohol, ethyl, etc. 10% aq.
Allylglycidylether, 0.25% MEK
Amethocaine, 5% pet.
p-Aminoazotoluene, 1% pet. or MEK
p-Aminobenzoic acid and esters, 5% pet.
p-Aminodiethylaniline, 1% pet.
Aminodiphenylamine 0.25% pet.
p-Aminophenol, 2% pet.
p-Aminosalicylic acid (PAS), 2% pet.
Ammoniated mercury, 2% pet.
Ammonium persulfate, 1% aq. (not
  stable)
Ampicillin, 5% aq.
Anethole, 2% alc. or pet.
Aniline, 1% pet.
Aniline dyes, 5% pet.
Anthraquinone, 2% pet.
Arnica tincture of, 20% alc.
Arylsulfonamide formaldehyde resin,
  10% acet.
Aureomycin, 5% pet.
Azo dyes, 1% pet. or MEK

Bacitracin, 20% pet.
Balsam of Canada, 25% pet.
Balsam of pine, 20% MEK
Balsam of spruce, 20% MEK
Balsam of tolu, 10% alc.
Beeswax, 30% pet. and olive oil ana.
Benzalkonium chloride,
  0.1%–0.01% aq.
Benzaldehyde, 5% pet. or 10% alc.
Benzetone chloride, 0.1% aq.
Benzidine, 1% MEK
Benzocaine, 5% pet.
Benzoyl peroxide, 2% pet. (not stable)
Benzyl alcohol (phenylcarbinol),
  5% pet.
Benzyl cinnamate, 5% pet. or 10% alc.
Bergamot oil, 2% pet.
Beryllium chloride, 1% aq.
Bisphenol A, 1% acet.
Butylacrylate, 0.5% pet.
Butulated hydroxyanisole (BHA), 2%
  pet.
Butulated hydroxytoluene (BHT), 2%
  pet.
p-t-Butylcatechol, 1% pet.
n-Butylglycidylether, 0.25% MEK
p-t-Butylphenol, 2% pet.
p-t-Butylphenol formaldehyde, 2% pet.

Captan, 0.1% pet.

123

Carbamide-formaldehyde, 10% pet.
Carbowax, as is
Cassia, oil of, 2% pet.
Cedarwood oil, 10% pet.
Cetylalcohol, 30% pet. and olive oil ana.
Cetylpyrimidine, 0.1% aq.
Chloramine, 0.5% aq.
Chloramphenicol, 5% pet.
Chlorhexidine, 0.5% aq.
Chloroacetamide, 0.1% aq.
Chloroacetophenone, 0.1% alc.
p-Chloro-m-cresol, 1% pet.
Chloroquine sulfate, 5% aq.
p-Chloro-m-xylenol, 1% pet.
Cincaine, 5% pet.
Cinnamic acid, 1% pet.
Cinnamic alcohol, 1% pet.
Cinnamic aldehyde, 1% pet.
Citral, 2% pet.
Citronella, oil of, 2% pet.
Cloves, oil of, 2% pet.
Coniferylbenzoate, 2% pet.
Copper sulfate, 1% aq.
Corticosteroids, use conc. and 10 times, pet.
Coumarin, 10% 0.0.
n-Cresylglycidylether, 0.25% MEK
Cyclohexyl-carbodiimide, 0.1% pet.

Dammar resin, 20% alc. or pet.
Diaminodiphenylmethane, 0.5% pet.
Diazodiethylanilinechloride, 2% pet.
Dibucaine, 5% pet.
Dibutylphthalate, 5% pet.
N,N'-Dibutyl-p-phenylenediamine, 1% pet.
Dichloro-hydroxy-quinoline, 5% pet.
Dichloronitrobenzene, 0.1% acetone
Dichlorophene (dihydroxydichlorodi-phenyl-methane), 1% pet.
Diethylaminosalicylate, 2% pet.
Diethylenediamine, 1% pet.
Diethylenetriamine, 1% MEK or pet.
Diethyl-p-phenylenediamine, 1% pet.

Diethylstilbestrol, 1% alc.
Dihydrostreptomycin, 0.1% pet.
Dihydroxydichlorodiphenylsulfide, 1% alc.
Dihydroxydiphenyl 0.1% pet.
Dimethylaniline, 1% pet. or alc.
Dimethylthiourea, 1% pet.
Dinitrophenylaniline, 1% pet.
Dioctylphthalate, 5% pet.
Dioctyl-p-phenylenediamine, DOPD, 2% pet.
Dioxane, 1% aq.
Dipentamethylenethiuramsulfide, 2% pet.
Dipentene, see Limonene
Diphenyl-methane-4, 4´-diisocyanate (MDI), 1% acet.
Diphenyl-p-toluidine, 2% pet.
Dipholatane, 0.1% pet.
Dithiocarbamates, 2% pet.
Di-o-tolylbiguanidine, 2% pet.
Dodecylgallate, 1% pet.
Dyes, organic, 2% pet.

Eosin, 50% pet.
Epichlorhydrin, 0.1% alc.
Epinephrine, 1% aq.
Epoxy resin, 1% acetone
Epoxy diluents (reactive), 0.25% MEK
Epoxy hardeners, 1 and 0.1% aq. or acet.
Erythromycin, 1% pet.
Essential oils, 1% pet.
Ethoxyquin, 1% ol. oliv.
Ethyleneoxide, 0.01% aq.
Ethylenediamine-HCl, 1% pet.
Ethylhexyl-acrylate, 0.5% pet.
Eucalyptus, oil of, 2% pet.
Eucerin, as is
Eugenol, 2% pet.
Explosives, 1% pet.
Fluorescein, 10% pet.
Fuchsin, 1% pet. or alc.

Gentamycin, 20% pet.

Geraniol, 5% pet.
Glutaraldehyde, 1% aq. (not stable)
Glycerolmonostearate, 30% pet.
Gold: K-dicyanoaurate, 0.05% alc.

Halogenated hydroxybenzoic acid
  esters, 5% pet.
Halogenated hydroxyquinolines,
  5% pet.
Halogenated salicylanilides, 1% MEK
Hardening agents, 0.1–1.0% aq. or acet.
Helenin, 0.1% pet.
Hexamethylenetetramine, 2% pet. or aq.
Hexylresorcinol, 2% pet.
Hydrazine, hydrate or sulfate, 1% pet.
  or aq.
Hydroquinone, 1% pet.
Hydroquinone-monobenzylether,
  1% pet.
Hydroxybenzoic acid esters, 5% pet.
Hydroxycitronellal, 1% pet.
Hydroxyquinolines, 5% pet.

Iodine, 0.1% alc.
Irgasan DP300, 0.5% aq.
Isocyanates, 0.1% acet.
Isoeugenol, 1% pet.

Kanamycin, 20% pet.

Lanolin, as is
Laurel, oil of, 2% pet.
Laurylgallate, 0.1% pet.
Lavender, oil of, 2% pet.
Lemon, oil of, 2% pet.
Lemon grass, oil of, 2% pet.
Lidocaine (Xylocaine), 2% pet.
d-Limonene (dipentene), 2% pet.

Malathion, 1% aq.
Maneb, 2% pet.
Melamine-formaldehyde, 10% alc.
2-Mercapto-6-nitrobenzothiazole,
  2% pet.

Mercury metal, 0.1% pet.
Merthiolate, 0.1% pet.
8-Methoxypsoralen 0.001% alc/aq.
Methyldichlorobenzene sulfonate, 0.1%
  pet.
Methylmethacrylate, 2% pet.
Methylol-chloracetamide, 0.5% pet.
Methyl orange, 2% pet.
Methyl-p-toluene sulfonate, 0.1% pet.
Methyl salicylate, 2% pet.
Metol(methyl-p-aminophenol sulfate),
  2% aq.
Mirbane oil, 10% O.O.
Monobenzylether of hydroquinone,
  1% pet.

α-(and β-)Naphthol, 0.1% pet. or 1% alc.
Naphtylamine, 2% alc.
Neroli, oil of, 2% pet.
Nipagins, see Hydroxybenzoic acid
  esters
Nitrofurazone, 1% pet.

Octylgallate, 0.1% pet.
Optical whiteners, 0.1–1% pet.
Orange, oil of, 2% pet.

Parabens, see Hydroxybenzoic acid
  esters
Penicillin, orig. solution
Pentachlorophenol, 1% alc.
Pentadecylcatechol, 0.1% pet.
Peppermint, oil of, 2% pet.
Percaine, 5% pet.
Peroxides, organic, 1% pet.
Phaltan, 0.1% pet.
Phenolic resin, 5% pet.
Phenothiazines, 1% pet.
Phenylcarbinol, see benzylalcohol
Phenylethanol, 5% pet.
Phenylglycidylether, 0.25% MEK
Phenylmercuric acetate, 0.01% aq.
Phenyl salicylate (Salol), 1% pet.
Phosphorsesquisulfide, as is

Photographic chemicals, 1% aq.
Phthalates, 5% pet.
Picric acid, 1% aq.
α-Pinene, 15% olive oil
Piperazine, 1% pet.
Piperazine derivatives, 5% aq.
Pitch, 5% pet.
Platinum chloride, 0.1% aq.
Polyethylene glycol, 1% alc.
Polymyxin B, 3% pet.
Potassium persulfate, 5% aq.
Probantheline bromide, 5% pet.
Propolis ointment, as is
Propylene glycol, 1 and 10% aq.
N-iso-Propyl-N-phenyl-PPD,
    0.1% pet.
Pyrethrum, 2% pet.
Pyrocatechol, 2% or aq.
Pyrogallol, 1% pet. or aq.

Quaternary ammonium salts, 0.1% and
    0.01% aq.
Quinine, 1% aq.

Resorcinol, 2% pet. or alc.
Resorcinol monobenzoate, 2% pet.
Retinoic acid, see Vitamin A acid
Rosin, see Colophony
Rubber chemicals, 2% pet.

Saccharin, as is
Salicylaldehyde, 2% pet.
Sodium diethyldithiocarbamate,
    2% pet.
Sorbic acid, 5% pet. or aq.
Spearmint, oil of, 2% pet.
Storax, oil of, 2% pet.
Storax, 2% pet.
Streptomycin, 0.1–1% aq.
Sulfonamides, 5% pet.
Sulfur, 1% pet.

Tall oil, 10% pet.
Tars, 5% pet.

Terramycin, 3% pet.
Tetracyclines, 5% pet.
Thiamine, 10% aq.
Thimerosal, 0.1% pet.
Tobacco, as is
p-Toluenediamine, 2% pet.
p-Toluidine, 2% pet.
Trichlorocarbanilide, TCC, 2% pet.
Tricresyl phosfate, 10% MEK
Triethanolamine, 2% aq.
Triethylenetetramine, 0.5% aq.
Trinitroanisol, 1% pet.
Trinitrophenol, 1% aq.
Trinitrotoluene, 1% pet.
Tylosin tartrate, 5% aq.

Urea-formaldehyde, 10% pet.
Usnic acid, 1% pet.

Vanilla, as is
Vanillin, 10% pet.
Venice turpentine = larch turpentine,
    20% pet.
Vitamin A acid(retinoic acid),
    0.005% alc.
Vitamin B_1, 10% pet.
Vitamin B_6, 10% pet.

Wood tars, 5% pet.

Xanthocillin, 10% pet.
Xylocaine, 2% aq.

Zineb, 2% pet.
Ziram, 2% pet.
Zirconium, sodium zirconium lactate,
    0.1% aq. intraderm. (Granuloma
    after weeks)

22.4 Products for testing

Use the actual batch of patients' products

Adhesive tape, as is
Ballpoint pen, dye, as is
Carbon paper, as is, wetted with acetone
Cleansers, do not test
Cosmetics, as is (some are irritants)
Cutting oil, 5% and 50% aq.
Diesel oil, do not test
Drilling oil, as is and 50% olive
  oil
Dye, food, as is and 2% pet.
Enzymes in detergents, do not test
Floor polish, do not test
Food, as is
Fruit (orange, citrus peel), as is
Furniture polish, 10% and 50% pet.
Glue, 1–20% aq., acetone, alc. or pet.
Hair dye preparation, 10% pet.
Hair lotion, 50% alc.
Hand lotion, as is and 50% pet.
Leather, test with extracts
Lubricating oils, as is and 50% olive oil
Mascara, 50% pet.
Metal, do not test

Nail polish, as is (after evaporation)
Oils, 5 and 50% ol. oil
Ointment, pharmaceutical, as is
Paints, as is and 10% and 50% pet. or
  water
Perfume, as is and 10% alc.
Permanent waving solution, do not test
Pesticides, 1% aq. or acetone
  (cholinesteras inhibitors 0.1%)
Petrol, do not test
Photographic chemicals, 1% and
  10% aq.
Photographic papers, as is
Plants, flower, stem, leaf, bulb, (see 4.14)
Plastics, hardeners, 0.1–1% aq. or
  acetone
Plastics, monomers 1–5% acetone
Printing sheets, as is
Rubber, as is
Textiles, as is
Thinner, 50% acetone
Wood, dry dust and 10% pet. (see 4.14)

Many products brought by patients are irritants. Open test and patch test with two or three concentrations should be performed. Many give false negative reactions, if possible, ingredients should be tested, e.g. preservatives in paint, glue, cosmetics, topical medicaments, oils.

22.5 Photo patch test substances

p-Aminobenzoates, 5% pet.
Bithionol, 1% pet.
Chloro- and bromo-salicylanilides, 0.5% pet.
Chlorosalicylamide, 1% alcohol or pet.
Chlorpromazines, 0.1% pet.
Dichlorophene, 1% pet.
Dimethylthiourea, 1% pet.
Fentichlor, 1% pet.
Hexachlorophane, 1% pet.
Lichens, as is
Musk ambrette, 5% pet.
Phenothiazines, 1% pet.
Quindoxin, 0.1% pet.
Quinine, 1% pet.
Sulfonamides, 5% pet.
Tricarbanilide (TCC), 1% pet.

Index

There are no page references to the lists of test substances 22.1–22.5

131

135